Medical Choices

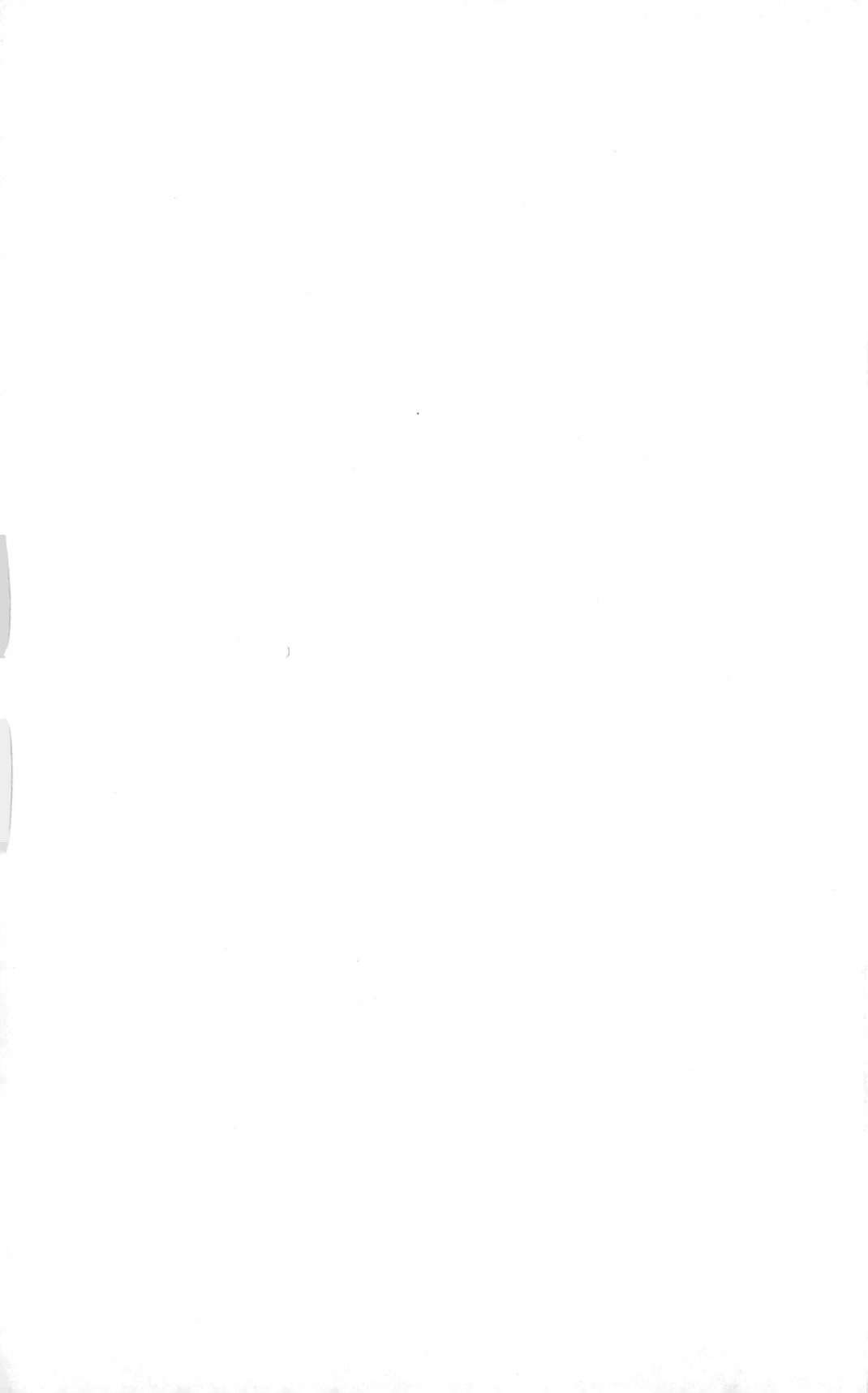

Medical Choices

Donald V. Gawronski, Ph.D.

Authors Choice Press
San Jose New York Lincoln Shanghai

Medical Choices

Authors Choice Press
an imprint of iUniverse, Inc.

For information address:
iUniverse, Inc.
5220 S. 16th St., Suite 200
Lincoln, NE 68512
www.iuniverse.com

This work makes no claim or endorsement for any health treatment. Make any
medical decisions in consultation with a qualified medical practioner

ISBN: 0-595-22232-3

Contents

PREFACE

Interest in the health movement, and in particular, alternative approaches in health care treatment, led to my being in frequent contact with individuals who were promoting a variety of health and nutritional products. Some of these individuals were quite knowledgeable; unfortunately, many were not. Only a scant few possessed a global knowledge of the health care industry.

This observation led me to a determination of the health care knowledge base of individuals who were not in the business of marketing health care products. The results were the same. Americans, it appears, know little about health care, relying on a quick technological fix whenever the occasion demands it, and know even less about how the megalithic health care industry operates. Not that information is unavailable, for it most certainly is. The newsletters of a number of national organizations regularly contain informative articles on health related issues. Some of this information even creeps into the mainstream press, although not usually in its original form and content. Individual, organizational, and governmental websites dealing with health related issues abound. But Americans who seek to discuss such issues are cast aside, viewed as "kooks" or alarmists. Disease, suffering, and dying are not pleasant topics, and are best avoided. Perhaps many Americans believe that by ignoring them they will go away.

I came to the conclusion that this little book needed to be written (whether it would be read or not was another issue). Many individuals, I believe, have need of some kind of guide to navigate them through the health care maze, and at one time, I even considered "Navigating the Medical Maze" as a title for the book, but discarded it as being misleading. So I wrote this book for a general audience, covering basic issues with as much brevity as possible without sacrificing meaning, and with every effort to avoid a scholarly or pedantic approach.

Most writing endeavors are group efforts. Although there may be but one author, many individuals influence, offer suggestions, and perhaps might even become actively involved in editing or reviewing. Certainly this is true respecting academic writing, but such was not the case for this effort. During the writing phase of *Medical Choices,* there was but one constant, and this was my wife. Pat, who is possessed of a deep interest in the subject matter contained in the text, as well as many of the issues raised. Having read heavily in the general areas of health and nutrition, she always seemed to have enough information to steer me in the right direction whenever I became rudderless. Further, her extensive library of health related books was put to good use. And she read and commented on the entire manuscript. So a special thanks and acknowledgement goes to Pat.

A portion of the manuscript was read by Mitchell Lover, who took time out from his busy schedule of running a health products marketing company to do so, and to Carol Keppler, who operates her own health products manufacturing and marketing company, whose detailed reading of the later chapters in the book led to the correction of some misstatements. Thanks to you both. Your time is valuable and you gave freely of it.

The title of the book posed a problem, given the topics of the various chapters. I bounced titles off of friends and neighbors and nothing seemed to fit. The actual title was suggested by my chiropractor, Stephen Grunfeld, D.C., who, after I outlined the various chapters in the book, took half a nanosecond to come up with "Medical Choices." Your contribution is appreciated; a book has to have a title.

All writing projects require technical assistance, especially due to the manner in which publishing is conducted today. My first book involved a typewriter, galley proofs, page proofs, and extensive editorial assistance. All of this is gone. Word processing and a radically changed way of conducting the publishing business are the culprits. Central to a contemporary writing endeavor is the presence of a word processing wizard. To Trinity DeJong, who aided me on a previous writing project, thank you again, for your technical help in preparing this material for submission.

And to anyone else who may have helped along the way, whether you realized it or not, you have my appreciation.

DVG   Scottsdale, Arizona

INTRODUCTION

This book is written for the health conscious layperson. It is intended to serve as a general introduction to the modern medical system, and how it became what it is. It does not suggest cures or endorse specific medical systems. Medical decisions are the responsibility of the individual in consultation with their chosen health care professional.

There is hardly a day that goes by without there being some article in the newspaper or news item on television dealing with a health related issue. Some are presented as positive by the media: a new wonder drug approved, or another exotic surgical procedure performed. Many others are clearly negative: an FDA attempt to curtail freedom of health choice, an insurance company or HMO denying coverage, the spiraling cost of pharmaceuticals, or another iatrogenically induced adverse event. How do all these related yet conflicting issues fit together? Modern health care appears to be both blessing and curse.

A growing number of individuals are becoming increasingly concerned about the quality, accessibility, and affordability of health care in America. There exists a crisis in confidence in the medical system. A national movement consisting of individuals seeking to take control over their own health is underway. This movement is taking many forms, ranging from exercise programs, diet, life style changes, the taking of nutritional supplements, preventive medicine, and various forms of alternative medicine. An increasing number of health care consumers are seeking, for a variety of reasons, treatment that is outside mainstream medicine, suggesting a growing lack of confidence in the medical establishment.

Scores of companies have arisen to meet the demands of the new health care market, offering a variety of nutritional and natural supplements. Some of these companies make use of the multi level marketing format to distribute their products, an approach wherein people tell other people, share their stories, present anecdotal evidence, and some scientific information. It is a populist approach, rooted in the egalitarian traditions of American culture, but clearly in conflict with institutionalized medicine. Other companies market their products through traditional retail outlets. The number of "health food" stores and nutritional chains has mushroomed over the past several decades. Additionally, drug stores, grocery stores, and general merchandise stores have climbed on the bandwagon, introducing "health" or "nutrition" sections in their places of business. If you have purchased or used health care products from any of these sources, or have thought about doing so, you can profit from this book, whose purpose is to describe the complicated modern health care system as simply as possible.

The practice of medicine today is hardly recognizable from its humble beginnings in the days of Hippocrates. In the first two chapters we will survey the evolution of medical practice from earliest times to the contemporary era. Knowledge of the past is necessary for an understanding of the present, so the book will follow a general historical approach. Modern medicine is highly technical, complicated, oftentimes impersonal, institutionalized, very expensive, and certainly bewildering to many of the patients it treats. But this, it has been argued, is the price that must be paid for progress. The nineteenth century English philosopher, Herbert Spencer, defined progress as the movement from the homogeneous to the heterogeneous, from tribal society to urbanized society, from single cell organisms to the higher mammals, and from the simple to the complex. If one were to apply Spencer's definition of progress to medicine, then most emphatically there has been substantial progress.

For not only does there exist sophisticated medical technologies, powerful pharmaceuticals, and an inexorable march of scientific reductionism aimed at an inquiry into the very building blocks of life itself (the human genome/proteome project), but there also exists a veritable myriad of medical treatment options and a confusing array of medical practitioners consisting of the MD, DO, ND, NMD, HMD, DVM, DDS, DC, OD, ad infinitum. In addition to the numerous specialties clustered under these titles, there is a broad array of different medical systems, such as ayurvedic medicine, Chinese medicine, Islamic medicine, native American medicine, and a plethora of folk medicines, to name a few. One might partake of music therapy, hydrotherapy, aromatherapy, a host of nutritional therapies, herbal medicine, therapeutic massage, magnetic field therapy, Reiki, and various types of spiritual healing. Some of these treatment modalities are controversial, while others are not. It depends on who one asks. The list is exhaustive, but no critical thinker can summarily dismiss any of these modalities. Yet how does one make an intelligent choice concerning treatment?

It is seriously doubted if most individuals are fully aware of the number of treatment options and types of health care practitioners available to them. Many patients are locked within the confines of the modern HMO, wherein options are quite limited and rarely discussed. One of the goals of this book is to identify and define the various treatment options and types of health practitioners available, and to put them into some perspective relative to each other. At issue also is the development of the ability to know when to seek out the type of treatment appropriate for one's condition. In other words, how does one become an informed consumer.

All treatments outside of the field of allopathic or conventional medicine are today referred to as "alternative." In the United Kingdom the term is "complementary." The terms "integrative" or "blended" or "holistic" are entering the vocabulary. The term "alternative" implies an either/or relationship: allopathic medicine or another type of treatment. The more recent terms suggest a cooperative treatment, and seem to me to reflect the best possible approach. Since "alternative" is the most widely used term I will use it throughout this book, but the reader is to understand that I do not use the term within the context of the either/or scenario.

A major difficulty associated with alternative medicine lies in ascertaining which modalities are based on solid science and which are, borrowing the term coined by Carl Sagan, "pseudo science." It is to be noted that a department within the National Institute of Health was created in 1998 to investigate the efficacy of various alternative treatments.

A problem inherent in some natural treatments results from the inability to isolate the specific substances or elements responsible for a claimed effect. Exact cause and effect relationships cannot be established scientifically. The principle reason for this is that some natural approaches are based on synergistic action, yet the very process of scientific reductionism, wherein objects are broken down into their most elemental particles, renders observation of synergism impossible. Furthermore, some natural treatments involve the combined action of body, mind, and spirit. Science is incapable of evaluating this type of treatment.

Some natural approaches are based on clearly observable scientific principles. It was the determination of specific healing properties in herbs that led to the development of synthetic chemical compounds and the modern pharmaceutical industry. Quantum physics has observed and now accepts the principle of synergism. And a number of research projects have proven quantitatively the power of the mind in the healing process. Placebo effect is real, but how does it measure up with science?

There still remains the absolute tie of cause and effect. The testimonials and endorsements that claim "a general feeling of well being," or "increased energy and vitality," are quite subjective and extremely difficult to prove on a scientific basis, even though they may indeed be quite true. Anecdotal "proofs" are often used in support of the efficacy of alternative treatments, yet this remains soft data. Statistical data is much more trustworthy; having been used quite successfully in the war on tobacco use. But quantitative data, too, is subject to interpretation....or misinterpretation. The scientific approach is not foolproof.

The fact that a treatment has been around for thousands of years does not necessarily prove it is effective, as some have maintained. It is equally true that just because some ancient form of medical treatment was discarded or neglected for tens of centuries that it is invalid, especially since modern science may now be able to prove its efficacy. The resurgent interest in acupuncture is a case in point.

Another goal of this book is to make some sense and organization out of the countless varieties of alternative medicine, and to place alternative therapies in proper context with allopathic medicine. The intent is that the reader will be able to make grounded preliminary decisions leading to much more detailed study of specific medical approaches, or, at the least, know what questions to ask.

A major alteration in the practice of medicine occurred during the latter half of the twentieth century. Health care is no longer characterized by a one–on–one relationship between patient and physician that one time existed. In many instances the personal physician has given way to institutionalized and highly commercialized medicine. Health care in America has become big business. The CEO's of the nation's largest HMO's receive annual compensation packages in excess of $50 million, and sales of prescription drugs reached $145 billion as of 2000, an increase of over 400% during the 1990's. The astronomical sums of money involved in health care services raise serious concerns over the sacrificing or compromising of medical ethics at the altar of the money god.

Of considerable concern is who really decides on treatment—the physician (who should), HMO policy, the insurance company, or an FDA regulation. There is no question as to the reality of the growing influence of the determination of treatment by forces other than the treating physician. There also exists a serious erosion of the rights of the patient to pick the type of treatment he/she prefers. The modern medical establishment has become quite dogmatic, and dogmatism runs counter to the very principles of a democratic society, as well as the very science allopathic medicine espouses.

Modern medicine is characterized by the presence of giant insurance companies, hospital associations, pharmaceutical corporations, "self regulating" professional associations, and accreditation boards. Where does the individual patient stand in the mix? The presence of powerful and oftentimes competing groups inevitably leads to conflict, and conflict leads to litigation. An increasingly influential player in the medical game is the legal profession, and a likewise increasing percentage of healthcare dollars are in the form of attorney and court fees. A chapter in this book will be devoted to a discussion of institutional or organizational medicine and its impact on the delivery of quality health care.

Rising health care costs is another issue. There is no question that overall healthcare costs are skyrocketing, increasing on an average of twice the annual inflation rate. This can most certainly be attributed partially to exotic new medical procedures, elaborate diagnostic equipment and intensive testing, and the cost of bringing an approved pharmaceutical to market. Some of this cost is unavoidable. But modern allopathic medicine emphasizes treatment rather than prevention. "An ounce of prevention is worth a pound of cure." In strictly economic terms is the statement true or false?

Some of the costs attributed to legitimate and unavoidable procedures and services are either overstated or misrepresented. The pharmaceutical industry, for example, claims the high cost of drugs is due to the cost of research and the FDA approval process. Yet the pharmaceutical industry spends more on advertising its products to the public each year than it does on research.. The end result is a legitimatized drug culture. How many people do you know who do not regularly use prescription or over the counter drugs? Believe it or not, there are some people who use such substances very sparingly.

The one area of cost containment that is within the control of every individual is prevention. We may not be the absolute master's of our fates, but we can change the odds, for life is choices. Allopathic medicine is beginning to take the cue, to "discover" what naturopathic medicine has known all along, that is, that prevention is a far less invasive and costly process, again, fully recognizing that sometimes the invasive process is the only viable option. Some HMO's are now establishing "wellness" programs, some dental plans are offering one or two "free" checkups and cleanings annually. Regular utilization of such services constitutes a positive step and reduces the need for more invasive treatment and subsequent higher costs. But on a more basic level a fundamental behavior exists.

Sometime over the course of the last forty years Americans have delinked rights and responsibilities. Increasingly, someone or something else is responsible for one's behavior and the consequences of that behavior. We are wallowing in the "cult of victimization." If I do something stupid my grandmother is to blame. If I lead an absolutely unhealthy lifestyle, exotic intrusive medicine is given the responsibility of "curing" the outward effects of my transgressions, but not the true causes. Save me from myself! Of course, self–responsibility requires discipline, study, and behavioral modification. I seriously doubt if anyone reading this material does not believe it, but do you *know* it?

Another growing problem concerns the dissemination of medical information. Increasingly, newspaper articles, television reports, and health websites, are prepared or financed by commercial health interests, and are, in effect, more commercial than news story. The line between medical fact and advertisement has been blurred on a number of medical websites. The practice has spread to professional medical journal articles as well. Pharmaceutical companies or their agents ghostwrite supportive articles, and offer them to medical doctors to sign and submit to journals. While not technically illegal, the practice is of questionable professionalism. As of mid 2001 the editors of professional medical journals have pledged to exclude these articles from their publications. We shall see. Former President Clinton called for an end to the "veil of secrecy" with which the medical profession reputedly shrouds itself. These, and other issues, will be detailed in a chapter on the status of contemporary medicine.

A separate chapter will be devoted to the topic of phytomedicine, that is, healing effects derived from plant materials. In this chapter we will consider three major modalities: phyto nutrients, flower essences and aromatherapy or essential oils. The newest of these modalities, phyto nutrients, is solidly based on laboratory science. The utilization of the subtle energy of plants through flower essences is a slightly less recent but popular modality. The use of essential oils is one of the most ancient medical treatments. Utilizing the lifeblood essence of plants, this ancient knowledge was relegated primarily to the cosmetics industry until rediscovered in the twentieth century. Much of phytomedicine is being scientifically validated.

This is equally true of "energy" or "vibrational" medicine. So many significant advances have occurred in just the last few years, that this topic also is deserving of separate consideration. A growing number of thinkers believe that energy medicine is the medicine of the future, and quantum science will validate it. It will be resisted, and it will be delayed, but it will occur. Investment in the "old" precludes objective evaluation of the "new." Such is the march of progress.

The march of humanity is not entirely linear; it is an ebb and a flow. The ever changing present continually attempts to dissociate with or revise its past, only to rediscover its past through its obsession with redefining it. The most ancient of medical treatments are making a powerful comeback, strengthened by new understanding of the nature of physical reality, and armed with scientific validation.

And finally, there is a crisis in healthcare. Stupidity has been defined as doing the same thing that does not work over and over again. While certainly not accusing anyone of stupidity, I am strongly suggesting that we need to be far more global and far less dogmatic in our attempts to address our societal problems. Fundamental changes in the healthcare culture need to occur. In the final chapter of this work we will speculate on ways to make healthcare better, cheaper, and more effective.

Chapter One

History of Medicine: Ancient to Allopathic

There are two dominant, but apparently diametrically opposing views concerning the living conditions of early humans. One view celebrates early humanity living in harmony with nature, in excellent health, blessed with long life, and possessed of intuitive truth and wisdom. This view is depicted in the Scriptural Garden of Eden and in the folklore surrounding the romanticized "noble savage." The other view describes a life in which sickness, disease, strife, debilitation, ignorance, and brief lifespan are the norms. Both views are partially correct. Certain non technical societies, such as the Hunzas, have enjoyed long life and health (at least until recently), and native Americans were reputed to be relatively disease free prior to contact with Europeans. Yet it does appear as if the greater majority of humanity experienced a life considerably less than utopian.

Most certainly, external conditions played a major role in determining the living conditions of early humans. Geography, climate, and diet would all have been controlling factors. Also not to be discounted was the frequency of war, the conditions associated with war, and the consequent transference of indigenous diseases from one culture to another. Non technical societies are extremely vulnerable due to their inability to control or manipulate natural phenomena.

From ancient times forward humanity has first attempted to understand, and secondly, to control, the processes that influence quality of life. Yet early humans possessed scant knowledge of the physical laws that governed them. The little knowledge that they did possess was generally mixed with substantial portions of superstition. This was certainly true regarding their concepts on illness.

Pre Historical Views on Health and Sickness

Minor illnesses were viewed as natural—the normal state of affairs over which some control could be exercised. Over an extended period of trial and error, perhaps lasting for millennia, early humans gradually discovered treatments that appeared to alleviate certain symptoms. Most of these treatments derived from plants and herbs, while some came from less savory sources. These treatments were handed down through an oral tradition and eventually comprised that vast body of unofficial wisdom known as folk medicine.

Early humans were hardly scientific in their orientation, but interestingly, modern science has discovered that many of the chemical properties contained within these ancient remedies were, indeed, appropriate for the symptoms being treated. Many modern pharmaceuticals derive from, or are synthesized versions of, these early folk treatments. Proper diagnosis was another matter.

Ancient humans probably did not realize it, but they were utilizing the empirical approach, that is, by observation they determined that certain treatments seemed to work for certain conditions. The reasons why were both unknown and unnecessary; it was the results that mattered. The scientific approach, on the other hand, is very much concerned with discovering the "why" of phenomena. It seeks to discover, to dissect, to analyze, and to replicate the specific substance or substances responsible for the effects being observed. Some extremely notable discoveries have thereby resulted and the contributions of the scientific method cannot be minimized.

But the very act of observing disturbs what is being observed. And this prevents it from ever being seen in its natural state. The act of separating a substance into its most elemental components, known as scientific reductionism, destroys any synergistic action that might be responsible for the effects being observed. And science rejects what does not submit to scientific methodology.

Herein lies a major conflict between the allopathic and natural approaches to medicine. The latter knows empirically, by observation and by intuition. The former knows rationally, by the pure exercise of reason, and is intellectual. A recurring theme in world literature and philosophy has unsuccessfully attempted to resolve this conflict. Can there be truth for which there is no observable scientific foundation?

Early humans viewed major illnesses in a manner entirely different from minor illnesses.. They were believed to be the external manifestations of some unnatural power: a demonic possession or the actions of an angry or mischievous anthropomorphic god. It was also oftentimes believed that the afflicted person had their "spirit" removed by some supernatural force, and the spirit had to be found and restored for the patient to get better. For this the gods had to be appeased or the demons had to be driven away. Treatment for major illnesses included rituals, chants, incantations—many apparent superstitious and unfounded practices.

Modern researchers are not so quick to dismiss these primitive practices in their entirety. Perhaps through trial and error, the same process that produced folk medicine, the ancient ones had stumbled upon something else that seemed to work that they did not understand.

Today we understand something called placebo effect, the ability of the mind to effect results from a non existent medication simply because it believes it is receiving that medication. Perhaps in the misty eons of the primeval past, rituals and spells had their origins in attempts to create a positive attitude in the patient for receptivity of the belief that the ritual would work, the power being in the belief, not the ritual itself. What is voodoo?

And were chants nothing but hopeless mumbo–jumbo. Today we understand the role of sound (frequency) as a treatment modality—ultra sound to aid in the repair of damaged tissue, or sound waves used to disintegrate gallstones. We understand the role of sound in influencing psychological change in the individual, through the actual altering of body chemistry. What moods are conveyed by the sounds of polyphonic counterpoint (medieval church music), a Sousa march, a Beethoven symphony, or the latest rapper? Language evolved first from sound, and it was the sounds that possessed the meaning. And although some of the original nature of language persists, much of it is artificial as it is now the word and not the sound that conveys the meaning.

Some medical centers are beginning to incorporate music therapy into their treatment programs. And most certainly music and chanting have played a major role in many major religious belief systems. Perhaps, without realizing it, ancients were the first holistic healers, again not knowing why what they did actually worked. There existed a blending of approaches in the craft of the shaman, the sorcerer, the oracle, and the witch.

But let us not make the error of giving too much credit to early humanity. Some of their treatments were bizarre and quite harmful. Primitives appear to have performed a form of surgery known as trepanning. Anthropologists have discovered that this practice existed throughout the ancient world, including the western hemisphere. Trepanning involved drilling a hole in one's skull, presumably to allow the evil spirit (disease) to escape, or to provide an entrance for the spirit to return (how the spirit managed to get out without a hole but needed one to get back in apparently was of no concern). Lest we be too critical of these beliefs recall that blood letting was the general treatment for many maladies not too long ago. One can only conjecture on what medical practitioners of the future might have to say about some of the treatments currently in use. Our practices are limited by our current level of understanding.

Most of our knowledge concerning early medical beliefs and practices is derived from anthropological study or from oral traditions that were eventually chronicled in the great religious scriptures of the world or the few surviving epic sagas. The first written record of medical practices obviously had to await the development of written language, and it is found in Babylonian clay tablets dating from around 3000 B.C. The later Code of Hammurabi, a codification of some 282 laws, and credited to a king by that name who ruled from 1792–1750 B.C., contains a number of references to surgical procedures, physicians fees, penalties for failure to cure (some were quite extreme), and two references to veterinarian surgeons.

The Ancient World

The *Epic of Gilgamesh*, long an oral tradition that was eventually chronicled around 1900 B.C., is a story of a Sumerian king seeking immortality. He hears of an unspecified plant growing at the bottom of a river that reverses the aging process. He eventually finds the plant, but while distracted, snakes eat the plant and obtain its benefits. The continual rejuvenation (immortality) of the snakes is evidenced by the regular shedding of their skins—an interesting interpretation of the origin of skin shedding. The Epic also makes several references to the burning of incense.

No substantive medical information has been derived from the Mesopotamian world, but such was hardly the case with Egypt. Hieroglyphs refer to the physician, Imhotep, who dates from the reign of Pharaoh Zoser (2980–2900 B.C.), builder of the famed step pyramid at Sakkara. Some surviving papyrus dates from 3000 B.C., and lists treatments, incantations, and various remedies. Yet much more can be deduced from the practice of embalming, and equally from the objects that would be found in the tombs of the pharaohs.

Egyptians believed that they had to take their possessions with them for use in the next life. So all they valued and deemed essential in the next world was packed into their burial chambers. Significant was the large number of vessels containing oils, many still in liquid form, some contained within gums and waxes. Some 350 such vessels were found in King Tut's tomb. Frankincense, often burned as an incense in honor of the god Ra, myrrh, regularly offered to the moon, and sandalwood, a principle ingredient in the embalming process, were the most commonly discovered oils.

The oldest known text of book length is the *Papyrus Ebers*, a 68 foot long, 12 inch wide scroll that provides an historical record of the medical beliefs and practices of the preceding two thousand years. Written in hieratic, a more fluid form of hieroglyphic, its black and red inks remain well preserved. The original papyrus has been sliced into pages and is on permanent view in the University of Leipzig library.

The *Papyrus Ebers* lists 811 prescriptions, ranging from single substances to combinations containing as many as 37 ingredients. Plants, oils, animal parts, human parts, insects, excrement (of all kinds), an infinite variety of beers, and various minerals, were used. Concoctions to treat skin ailments, dandruff, abcesses, and even smelly feet, were included. A number of surgical procedures were described. Over 700 "drugs" are mentioned. Well worth reading as an historical curiosity, the *Papyrus Ebers* most certainly bears witness to the blending of empiricism and superstition in the ancient world.

One of the earliest aromatics used by the Egyptians was a substance known as kyphi. First burnt as an offering to the god Ra, it was eventually used as a household air freshener, perfume, and in time, as a medicine. Plutarch's description of the effects of kyphi suggest that it possessed narcotic properties. Allegedly it consisted of sixteen ingredients, but modern analysts are not agreed on what they were.

Due to historical connectedness, Egyptian medical practices were inter-twined with the early Hebrew tradition. The *Old Testament* is replete with references to herbs, plants, and oils, though it is lacking in direct medical information. Still, there are references to diet and hygiene that were based on principles that continue to possess validity to the present day.

Early Eastern Medicine

Some of the earliest medical treatises come from the East. Around 2000 B.C. Indian sacred writings known as the *Vedas* proposed a system of med-icine known as Ayurveda, which would maintain its dominance for over 1200 years. A holistic approach, Vedic medicine utilized numerous herbs and incantations. Ayurvedic medicine continues to be practiced to the present day and will be discussed in some detail in the chapter on alterna-tive medicine.

Brahmanistic medicine would hold sway in the Hindu world from around 800 B.C. to 1200 A.D. Hindu religious beliefs prohibited dissec-tion of the human body, so little was known of the inner workings of the body (interestingly, Egyptians, with all their embalming activities, were equally lacking in this regard). Brahmanistic medicine developed stan-dardized diagnostic procedures, classified diseases (over 1100 of them, most of which were various types of fever), prescribed diet, a variety of medicines, and included a fair portion of magic. One surviving text lists 760 medicinal plants. Medical treatments included enemas, purgatives, inhalations, blood letting, and cupping. The Hindus developed a number of surgeries, and detailed the procedures and instruments used. As with most surgeries well into the nineteenth century, the anesthetic of choice was alcohol.

Chinese medicine developed independently of any outside influences. Tradition places its origins with the real or mythical Fu His around 3000 B.C. Numerous medical texts have survived, the most influential of which is *Nei Ching.* Balance is key to traditional Chinese medicine to the present day. To be healthy the body must be balanced in its Yang and Yin forces, Yang being associated with masculinity, activity, light, and heaven, and Yin being associated with femininity, passivity, darkness, and earth. The major procedure used for determining this balance was pulse taking, an elaborate process requiring the taking of ten minute pulses at three different levels each, at various locations of the body. The process could take many hours to complete. Diagnosis also included examining the tongue and listening to the voice.

Chinese pharmacology embraced over 1000 herbal substances, utilized according to "signature theory," that is, using herbs and plants that were shaped like various parts of the body or its organs to treat that particular area. Some herbs were named after the body organs they resembled, or for the condition they were used to treat. Those names have survived to the present day. Hydrotherapy, moxibustion, and acupuncture rounded out the treatment options. Immunization for smallpox was used by around 400 B.C., but it is highly unlikely that the Chinese understood how, or even if, the process worked. This knowledge was repudiated in the West until the early eighteenth century (because of its pagan origins), by which time some of the beliefs of the medieval church had been successfully challenged.

Ginseng was the most popular plant (actually it was the root that was most desired) used in China. The most prized, and therefore the most expensive ginseng, was the root that most closely resembled the human form—signature theory. In traditional circles this belief continues to the present day.

Japanese medicine was strongly influenced by the much older Chinese culture. Japanese medical students learned their craft in China, and the first known Japanese medical text, *Ishinho,* dating from the latter part of the tenth century, fully reflects the Chinese medical thinking of that era. The late sixteenth and early seventeenth centuries witnessed the publication of numerous medical treatises written by the celebrated Japanese physicians, Dosan and Tokuhun. Dosan is reputed to be the world's first documented gereontologist.

When Asia came into contact with the West in the sixteenth century, China and Japan embarked on different courses. China rejected all things western, and successfully closed its borders to the West until the results of the Sino–Japanese War (1895) revealed its tremendous vulnerability. Japan, on the other hand, had made a conscious decision to learn what it could from the West, while simultaneously preserving its unique culture.

It was European missionaries who introduced western style medicine to Japan, and by the eighteenth century, the Japanese had successfully translated all known western medical texts. A deliberate national effort was undertaken to adopt western medicine. In 1859 a western style medical school was established, and Japan began making advances and discoveries along the lines of their western colleagues.

The Greek Period

Meanwhile major developments were pending around the Aegean Sea. Minoan and early Greek medicine was dominated by superstition and by belief in vengeful anthropomorphic gods, that is, until the appearance of Hippocrates. Much concerning Hippocrates is legend. He is reputed to have lived around 460–377 B.C., and to have written 60–70 medical texts, but this is not historical fact. Surviving medical text of his time period may have been written by him, perhaps by others, or perhaps he chronicled what others had written before him. A youthful contemporary of Hippocrates was Plato who, in his writings, later referred to Hippocrates as a very distinguished physician. A student of Aristotle's by the name of Meno, in his history of medicine, credited Hippocrates as the source of his medical knowledge. Aristotle, himself, wrote that Hippocrates was known as the "Great Physician."

Hippocrates rejected superstition. All diseases, he believed, must have an external cause, and it was the function of the physician to determine that cause and then help the body to heal itself. Very temperate in his use of medicines, Hippocrates may well have been the first naturopath. But he is best known for the code of ethics that bears his name, a code most scholars now believe he did not author. It is here included in its entirety so that the reader may personally decide how closely it reflects the version of the code approved by the American Medical Association.

I swear by Apollo the physician, and Aesculapius, and Health, and All–heal, and all the gods and goddesses, that, according to my ability, and judgment, I will keep this Oath and this stipulation—to reckon him who taught me this Art equally dear to me as my parents, to share my substance with him, and relieve his necessities if required; to look upon his offspring in the same footing as my own brothers, and to teach them this art, if they shall wish to learn it, without fee or stipulation; and that by precept, lecture, and every other mode of instruction, I will impart a knowledge of the Art to my own sons. And those of my teachers, and to disciples bound by a stipulation and oath according to the law of medicine, but to none others, I will follow that system of regime which, according to my ability and judgment, I consider for the benefit of my patients, and abstain from whatever is deleterious or mischievous. I will give no deadly medicine to any one if asked, nor suggest any such counsel; and in like manner I will not give to a woman a pessary to produce abortion. With purity and with holiness I will pass my life and practice my Art. I will not cut persons laboring under the stone, but will leave this to be done by men who are practitioners of this work. Into whatever house I enter, I will go into them for the benefit of the sick, and will abstain from every voluntary act of mischief and corruption; and, further from the seduction of females or males, of freemen and slaves. Whatever, in connection with my professional practice or not, in connection with it, I see or hear, in the life of men, which ought not be spoken of abroad. I will not divulge, as reckoning that all such should be kept secret. While I continue to keep this Oath unviolated, may it be granted to me to enjoy life and the practice of the art, respected by all men, in all times! But should I trespass and violate this oath, may the reverse be my lot!

Hippocrates advocated a daily aromatic bath and scented massage. He also urged the burning of aromatic plants in the streets of Athens to prevent the spread of the plague, a practice to be utilized by medieval Europeans for the same purpose. The Greeks believed in living in a highly scented world. All pleasant smells were believed to be of divine origin.

The major Greek contribution to western civilization was rationality. Yet the path from superstition to reason was a long and arduous one. The Greek god of medicine was Aesciepius, who may have been an actual human healer who lived around 1200 B.C. But differentiation between gods and humans was sometimes quite vague in the ancient world.

The numerous temples dedicated to Aesciepius were very much like health spas, where people went to "incubate," meaning, to be cured by divine intervention. It was the philosophers who attempted to introduce sanity, who sought out rational causes for observed effects. But sometimes reason fared no better. The views of the fifth century B.C. philosopher, Empedocles, led to the "discovery" of the four humours, they being blood, bile, cholera, and melancholy. Lack of balance between the four humours was believed to cause ill health. Humours persisted well into early modern European history.

Although known primarily as a philosopher, Aristotle was also a keen student of the natural world. Son of a court physician to a Macedonian king, Aristotle became acquainted with Greek medical knowledge at a very early age. The latter part of his life was devoted to scientific inquiry, and subsequently, Aristotle is regarded as being a founding influence on the fields of comparative anatomy and on embryology.

The Roman Period

The Roman world, which eventually overtook that of the Greeks, absorbed Greek medical knowledge and practice. The Greek belief in daily baths, so ardently championed by Hippocrates, provides one telling example. Archeological evidence indicates a multitude of private and communal baths in the Roman world, and they were usually aromatic. The Greek center of medical training in Alexandria continued to be as much of a dominant force under the Romans as it had been under the Greeks.

Rome also absorbed much of Egyptian medical knowledge. Dioscorides wrote a medical treatise in the first century A.D. that became the vehicle for the transfer of Egyptian medical knowledge throughout Europe through the expansion of the Roman Empire. The work consisted of five parts, with one dealing exclusively with aromatics, again, displaying the influence of the Egyptians and Greeks on Roman culture.

Roman culture is best noted for its ability to build and organize, and it is through the exercise of these skills that Roman civilization made its contribution to the medical field. Rome was very good at making laws, and numerous laws were promulgated that dealt with public health issues. In sewerage disposal, public water supply, hospitals, public baths, and gymnasia, the Romans excelled. Yet their substantive medical knowledge came mainly from the Greeks.

Asciepiades proposed that the body was made up of tiny particles (the atomist theory of reality was originally proposed by Democritus in the fifth century B.C.), and that the disharmony of these particles is what causes illness. He proposed standard Greek treatments to restore this harmony: massage, diet, tonics, and so forth. Whether or not disharmonious particles were the root of illness was probably of no lasting significance. But Asciepiades did propose some rather enlightened views on mental illness. He proposed occupational therapy, music therapy, and exercise to mitigate some of the effects of mental illness.

In 30 A.D. Celsus wrote a survey of Greek medical practices that included all the standard surgical procedures of the day. But it was Galen in the second century A.D., who thoroughly cemented Greek medical practices to the West. A staunch believer in Hippocrates, who equally accepted the concept of the four humours, he nonetheless gained some insight in the cardio–vascular sphere. Sometimes being credited as the Father of Physiology, Galen learned a great deal about the human body while patching up gladiators. Later, as official physician to the Roman Emperor, he occupied much of his ample spare time studying physiology by inferring human anatomy from his dissection of primates (it was illegal in all cultures to dissect human remains before the modern era).

The Early Middle Ages

The disintegration of the Roman Empire in the West, which historians date as 476 A.D., ushered in the so–called Dark Ages. Europe was to undergo centuries of amalgamating Greek, Roman, Christian, and Germanic influences into what would eventually become European civilization. The prevailing paradigm embraced a providential view of history. This paradigm interpreted the world as a waiting room for eternity, wherein an active Divine Providence rewarded good and punished evil on the earthly plane. Ipso facto, the presence of disease was a divinely ordained punishment, and obviously deserved, since God was deemed to be just. Suffering became an entitlement; it earned an eventual place in heaven. To prevent suffering was to interfere in the workings of the Divine Plan. Yet at the same time Jesus had charged his followers to care for the sick.

Many saints were declared the patron benefactors of various earthly ailments. Medical treatment consisted mainly in praying to the saint who reputedly had particular interest in a certain part of the body or specific ailment, begging for intercession with God and forgiveness of the sins that were believed responsible for the malady.

Concurrently, some monasteries were busy copying and preserving ancient medical texts. In the West these manuscripts were translated into Latin; at a much later date they would be translated again into vernacular languages. In the East manuscripts were translated into Arabic, thereby providing a starting point for the transcendence of Islamic medicine.

The Birth of Islamic Medicine

The Eastern Roman Empire, or Byzantium, would last until 1453 A.D. Eastern Rite Christians, later termed Greek Orthodox, were considerably more tolerant than their western counterparts. Their paradigm included enjoying the world and its pleasures. The Islamic world was an eclectic world, consisting of a multiplicity of races, ethnicities, and religions. The cultural mix promoted free inquiry. Human achievements are only limited by the boundaries humanity places on itself. The Islamic world produced schools, hospitals, and numerous advances in medical science.

Early Islamic medicine arose around the city of Jundishapur. Originally a settlement of Greek prisoners, it eventually developed a medical school and a hospital. But it appears that Byzantine emperors were not entirely consistent. Periodically, they would close down their medical training centers and expel the Greek physicians in residence there. These refugees were given sanctuary in Junishapur, located in ancient Syria. There, Greek medical knowledge was brought into contact with that of India. After the

Islamic conquest of the region, the center was protected and nurtured, and became the prototype of Arabian medical training. Based on Hippocrates and Galen, repudiating superstition and emphasizing science, the center would feed the establishment of medical centers in Bagdad during the eighth century A.D.

This led to the development of the "House of Wisdom" in the ninth century when a concerted national effort scoured the eastern world in search of ancient manuscripts dealing with science and medicine. Many were discovered and translated, aiding in the explosion of Arab knowledge during the Middle Ages.

One of the earliest and most celebrated contributors to Islamic medicine was Rhazes, a Persian who died in 925 A.D. Credited with authoring 56 medical texts, his technique for distinguishing measles and smallpox was widely disseminated in the West. The first major Islamic surgical work was actually written in the West, in Arab Spain, by Albucasis. It was the final volume of a thirty volume medical work, indicating perhaps the amount of emphasis that was being placed on surgery at the time.

A contemporary, Avicenna (980–1037 A.D.),. is the recognized giant of Arab medicine. His *Canons of Medicine* was destined to become the principle medical text used in the West until the mid seventeenth century, and in the East, to an even later date. Proving the eclecticism of Arab culture, Avicenna was actually a Persian, while another great figure in Arab medicine, Maimonides, was a Jew. Maimonides was personal physician to Saladin, and authored *The Code of Maimonides*, a compendium of medical ethics highly esteemed in Jewish culture. Maimonides wrote in Hebrew, but much of his work was translated into Latin.

Alchemy was widely studied in the Arab world, its origins being attributed to Jabik ibn Hayyan in the late tenth century. Numerous substances and compounds were discovered, and their names to the present day reflect their Arab origin. A case could be made crediting the Arabs with the invention of pharmacology. Their medical knowledge, based on a foundation of Egyptian and Greek achievements, was enhanced by a tremendous increase in botanical knowledge, a byproduct of Islamic geographical expansion. The Arabs definitely possessed knowledge of distillation, crystallization, and sublimation. These processes were of major importance in the preparation of oils, drugs, and extracts.

In the eleventh century Constantinus Africanus deserves major credit for translating Hippocrates, Galen, and Arab medical treatises into Latin. The twelfth century witnessed further translations of both medical and philosophical texts by way of Muslim Spain. This effort was led by Gerard of Cremona. Medicine was becoming a blending of classical tradition and Islamic advances within a Christian framework

That framework subordinated the physical to the spiritual; saving the soul took precedence over saving the body, and the Last Rites were more significant than medical treatment. The plagues that racked Europe were attributed to punishment for lust or caused by the Jews. So persecute the Jews and/or repent. Self flagellation was an excellent remedy. The most widely used medical remedy for the plagues was aromatic herbs and oils, and a few rational beings were even able to discern its true causes. Quarantines were introduced and somewhat enforced. The constant presence of death cast a macabre shadow on Europe. The symbol of the Grim Reaper is a product of the age.

Renaissance Medicine

Yet the learned men of the day, who were invariably clerics, were also precursors of the later "Renaissance man." A new spirit was awakening in Europe. The abortive Age of the Crusades was creating some unforeseen positive results for Europe. Contact with the Middle East had reacquainted Europe with its own rich past. The Arabs had preserved and added to that record of the past, whereas many early Christians had systematically destroyed whatever was labeled as being of "pagan" origins. Europe began to ameliorate its providential paradigm and began to uphold mankind for the sake of man, in a movement known as the Renaissance, or rebirth

The Renaissance began in the Italian city–states, but gradually its influences were felt throughout Europe. In southern Italy one immediate result was the appearance of the first European medical school, located at Salerno. Famous primarily because it was first, its appearance soon led to the establishment of more substantive institutions at Padua and Bologna in Italy, and at Montpellier and Paris in France. Spanning the end of the Renaissance era and the beginning of the Age of Enlightenment, the Royal College of Physicians and Surgeons was decreed for England and Scotland.

The Renaissance is best known for its accomplishments in art. Paradoxically, the zeal to create perfectly realistic human forms in painting, and particularly in sculpture, encouraged the study of human anatomy. Of note is Andrea Vesalius, anatomy professor at the medical school in Padua. Advances in anatomical knowledge had obvious positive effects on the practice of surgery. Ambrose Pare, arguably the father of modern surgery, replaced the common practice of cauterization (which often led to infection), with ligatures, which also had the effect of closing the wound and hastening the healing process.

During the twilight of the Renaissance there appeared Theophrastus von Hohenheim (1490–1541), the offspring of a country physician, and reputedly possessed of an extremely bombastic personality. Preferring to call himself Paracelsus, he became disenchanted with the study of medicine, traveled widely, and eventually took a job working in the mines at Tryol. There he became familiar with the chemical processes used to refine ore. Blending his earlier medical training with his newly acquired knowledge of ore processing, Paracelsus posited that if mineral substances could be used to refine other mineral substances from the mines, why could not the same process be used in the human body?

Rejecting the naturopathic views of Hippocrates, Galen, and Avicenna, whose works he publicly repudiated and burned, Hohenheim experimented with the application of chemical compounds and minerals to the human body. There are no known records of the results of his experiments, but Hohenheim succeeded in introducing the world to chemical medicine, a radical change. He is reputed to be the first to prescribe mercury to treat syphilis, which was of epidemic proportions and believed to have been spread by the sailors of Columbus. Mercury, or quicksilver, was quaksilber in German, and at the time, was being prescribed for a multitude of ailments, becoming the proverbial snake oil of its day. This over prescription gave rise to the term "quack."

Hohenheim marks a critical junction in the practice of medicine. From pre history up to around 1500 A.D., no physician utilized anything other than natural substances in treatment. After 1500, however, the natural healing tradition of Hippocrates and others would be maintained primarily by herbalists, who would continue the ancient dictum of placing "no harmful substance" in the body. Overwhelmingly, medicine would begin to march to the Hohenheim tune. There is no question that pharmaceuticals are much more powerful and fast acting than are natural substances, and generally more effective as well, The trade off concerns the side effects generally associated with synthesized drugs, and the resultant chain reaction. An additional concern is whether healing is being undertaken, or, are effects being masked and causes left intact. Modern drugs clearly can be lifesavers properly administered (see Chapter Eight).

The Expansion of Europe

In part the changes taking place in Europe were due to the geographical expansion of Europe. Contact with the New World brought medical disaster. Of the twenty original domesticated animals in the world, nineteen were from Eurasia, and only one from the New World, the llama. Much of human disease was acquired from animals (called zoonoses) by living with animals and in concentrated populations. Those Europeans who survived the many plagues that decimated Europe over the centuries both developed an immunity and became carriers of these diseases.

New World inhabitants had lived in relative isolation from Eurasia for thousands of years (there had been sporadic contact, for example, the Vikings) and were essentially disease free, except for the standard health issues arising out of growing population density. The Spanish conquest inadvertently wiped out 90 percent of the New World population with whom it came into contact during the sixteenth century. The culprits were influenza, smallpox, and measles. The decimated workforce was replaced with the importation of Africans as slaves, and this further complicated the issue. African diseases, notably malaria and yellow fever, were also brought to the New World, and affected Spaniard and indigenous population as well.

During the seventeenth century it was England and France who were the culprits, mainly in the northern reaches of North America, mainly by spreading smallpox. The worldwide intermixing of isolated populations created the greatest health crisis in world history, rearranged the populations of the continents, and practically destroyed New World indigenous peoples. Europeans initially traveled to the New World in very small ships, and came in limited numbers. Disease was their greatest weapon in conquering the New World.

And what they did to the New World they did to themselves. What was the source of the epidemic of venereal disease at the time is not known. In some way the long dormant spirochete was reawakened, perhaps aided by contact with new populations, perhaps not.

Worldwide conquest brought other developments. Hundreds of new plants were discovered in the New World, and eventually, through direct contact with the Far East. Opium was introduced from the East, tobacco from the West (it was considered a medicine at the time). Cinchona, or Peruvian bark, and regularly used in the New World, contains quinine, later proven effective in the treatment of malaria. Ipecacuanha, from

Brazil, was useful for the treatment of dysentery and was also used as an expectorant and an emetic.

The explosion of knowledge that was accompanying worldwide disaster was enhanced by an invention, the printing press, which made possible the widespread dissemination of knowledge. The printing press has been cited as the greatest invention of the second millennia. Aiding the process was the move to vernacular language. Latin had been the universal language of the intellectual elite; Greek ran a distant second. But writing in the vernacular was important for the popularization of knowledge. The beginning of the end of monopoly of information was itself a monumental event that would eventually lead to ideas of egalitarianism and democracy.

The European Enlightenment

The seventeenth and eighteenth centuries in Europe are known as the Age of the Enlightenment. The period opened with a number of discoveries and inventions that would make possible a more accurate inquiry into the nature of the physical world, for example., the microscope, the telescope, the pendulum clock. As the notables of the early movement uncovered hitherto unknown laws of nature, such as Isaac Newton's Three Laws, a wave of euphoria swept Europe, and culminated in a belief that simple laws governed everything; they merely had to be discovered. The universe was now viewed as mechanistic; scientific methodology became the only trusted process; Rene Descartes proposed that the human body was nothing more than a machine, and that the only thing that differentiated humans from animals was the existence of a soul. A contemporary, Thomas Hobbes, even repudiated the soul.

The work of Albrecht von Haller proved no help to the theological view. Noting that muscles responded to stimuli and nerves reacted to pain, he suggested some sort of mechanical function. Later experimentation by the Italians Luigi Galvani and Alessandro Volta solved the problem; it was electricity. The mechanistic view accounted for the differentiation of life forms as simply being a matter of the degree of development, with humans at the top of the scale. This could still be attributed to a Divine Plan. But the theorized mutation of specie due to environmental factors proposed by Erasmus Darwin, laid the foundation for the later monumental evolution theories advanced by his grandson, Charles Darwin. The Divine was being squeezed out of the equation.

The monumental work of William Harvey was the result of employing the new scientific methodology. His theories on the circulation of the blood were the results of laboratory experimentation, and not on speculation. Harvey's epochal theories were refined by the Italian, Marcello Malpighi, and later still, by Richard Lower, who made the connection between blood and air. In the eighteenth century, Lavoisier would discover how oxygen works in the body, through circulation and respiration.

Change does not occur on a continuum, but rather on a pendulum. Once a new idea or approach gains some receptivity, it inevitably is overly reacted to or overstated, and much unnecessary grief has to be endured before it finally settles appropriately. Such is the human condition and so it was with the mechanistic theory. Iatrophysicists attempted to explain the human body only in mechanistic terms, while iatrochemists viewed the body strictly as a series of chemical processes. One of the byproducts of scientific reduction is that with its emphasis on pursuing the minute parts, it sometimes forgets that what it is seeking is part of a whole. In the contemporary era we use the term "systems theory," that is, the study of the integration of the various parts to create the entire system.

Progress may well be defined as a movement from the simple to the complex, but there are always those who seek to react to growing complexity with increased simplicity. Such was the case with John Brown, who developed his "Brunonian System," a very simplistic view of medicine, and this at a time when science was in its ascendancy. There are only two diseases: strong and weak, and two treatments: stimulant and sedative, and two remedies: alcohol and opium. The more alcohol or opium used, the better it was believed would be the results. It is highly doubtful if anyone was healed thereby, but judging from the remedies used, they probably did not care. Brown also quantified health on a scale of 0–80, with 40 being homeostasis or health. How he came up with his numbers is another story.

An advocate of the "less is better" school, on the other hand, was Samuel Halneman, the founder of homeopathy (see Chapter Three). He proposed very small dosages of compounds whose effects mimicked the malady being treated. Homeopathic medicine is very much alive today, and constitutes a government regulated treatment modality.

The Birth of Eclecticism

Medical forms and practices were developing in other parts of the world, some of an indigenous nature, some the product of contact with the West. The bureaucracies that arose in the East, as far as medicine is concerned, maintained their status in society by claiming to safeguard that which was of divine origin. Eastern medicine claimed an unknown or forgotten origin that became dogma. Religiously held medical beliefs are very difficult to change, traditional beliefs only slightly less so. Throughout most the eastern world ancient beliefs have never been entirely sublimated by western scientific medicine.

No formal medical text appeared in India until the first century *Caraka Sambita* and the fourth century *Susruta Sambita*. The ayurvedic medicine advanced in these texts emphasized natural cures, but originally involved some surgery. References to surgery diminished over time, ostensibly due to the development of the Hindu caste system and its limitations on who could touch whom. India is a very large and diverse country. Its medical practices have been influenced by China, the world of Islam, and by the West, as well as its own indigenous belief systems. Ayurvedic was popular in northern India, while the southern part of the country seemed to prefer alchemy, astrology, and divination. Contact with Islam brought Yunani medicine, Arabianized Galen. Dutch and British colonization suppressed traditional medicine, replacing it with western style medicine. Urban, upper class Indians today prefer western medicine, while ayurvedic is preferred in rural areas and by the lower classes

Chinese medicine, like all things Chinese, revolves around the principle of orthodoxy; there are set ways of doing things. Confucius had proscribed the rules of bureaucratic behavior that survived into the early twentieth century. Chinese medicine is equally based on ancient orthodoxy. The *Inner Canon* and the *Canon of Problems* date from the origins of the Chinese nation, and were attributed to legendary figures. All formal healers were required to be thoroughly familiar with, and abide by, these two works. The first work cited was a general medical text; the second work described specific treatments. Chinese medicine emphasized needling, a broad term encompassing blood letting and acupuncture. The later *Divine Husbandsman's Materia Medica* catalogued drugs, arranging them from gentle and long term to strong and short term. And finally the *Treatise on Cold Damage Disorders* dealt with infectious fevers and their treatments. All treatment involved medicines.

Ancient Chinese beliefs held that sickness was punishment for offending ancestors or curses. Over time environment became the culprit. The world is made up of chi; life is concentrated chi, and death is the diminishing of chi. Chinese medicine concentrated less on the body and more on cosmic process. The dynamic process of ever changing chi is the yang and yin "opposites." The Chinese practice of acupuncture rests on the belief in chi, the blockage of which creates illness in the body. It is an ancient practice that has been gaining in popularity with the alternative medicine movement, and the more recent interest in vibrational or energy medicine, in part encouraged by advances in quantum physics.

By the beginning of the nineteenth century the working of the human body was generally understood. Most basic diagnostic equipment had been invented, and substantive examination procedures had been developed. The state was thereby set for a more scientific delving into the field of medicine.

Chapter Summary

- Though lacking a scientific basis, early humans developed a rudimentary medicine through trial and error.
- Practices long regarded as mere superstition are today being discovered to have some basis in fact.
- Papyri of ancient Egypt provide the earlier known written works on medical treatment.
- Archeological evidence in Egyptian tombs provide information on what was important for the next life. Oils and aromatics ranked high on the list.
- Surviving ancient texts from Asia emphasize herbology and the balancing of life forces.
- Of all Asian nations China was most successful in preserving its traditional medical beliefs.
- Hippocrates is regarded as the first naturopathic physician. His famous Oath has been edited massively by modern medical organizations.
- The Greeks emphasized scents, baths, massage, and the balance of body vital forces.
- The Romans absorbed Greek medicine to which they added public health law. Their sanitation and water systems were significant for the promotion of health.
- Medical knowledge languished in early Europe. Suffering was to be accepted as Divine punishment. The works of the classical period were deliberately destroyed since they were of pagan origin. Yet some preservation took place in various monasteries.

- Islam inherited, preserved, and enhanced Greek medicine. Arab medicine texts were introduced to Europe around the end of the first millennium.
- Islamic work in alchemy led to the development of pharmacology.
- The Crusades introduced Arab medicine and the Greek medical heritage to Europe, providing one aspect of the Renaissance.
- At the end of the Renaissance Hohenheim ended the centuries old tradition of treating only with natural substances. He is regarded as the founder of chemical medicine.
- European expansion resulted to worldwide health disaster, as European diseases were spread to indigenous populations who had no immunity.
- European expansion was also responsible for the discovery of numerous New World medicinal plants.
- The European Enlightenment challenged the religious hold on medical truth. The universe and the human body were henceforth viewed mechanistically.
- Homeopathy developed in reaction to the new chemical and mechanistic medicine.
- Early modern Asian medicine is characterized by orthodoxy, divine inspiration, and western influence.

Chapter Two

A History of Allopathic Medicine

The basic institutions of any society tend to reflect an underlying commonality. If a society is dominated by religion then religion permeates every aspect of life; if by a dogmatic political system, then a political agenda dominates. This underlying commonality constitutes a belief system, a filter through which reality is received and then interpreted. In the contemporary world we refer to this belief system as a paradigm.

Nineteenth Century Medicine

The nineteenth century opened in the immediate aftermath of the French Revolution, which, with its obliteration of the social, political, and economic systems of the past, did not rest content. Once the floodgates of change had been opened, all institutions, systems, and beliefs were vulnerable. Attacked they were, and a radically changed calendar, a revamped educational system, a new mode of dress, and a new national banking system were but a few consequences of this rampant change.

A completely new medical system was also a product of the French Revolution. The revolutionary climate had rendered it quite easy to discard any prevailing belief or practice, and more importantly, any established privilege. The old established medical order was one such privileged institution, but change, which rarely comes about without considerable resistance, was the order of the day.

One development concerned the replacement of the Church by the state as the primary institution for delivering medical care. Certainly this development was occurring in other European nations due to the widespread growth of nationalistic fervor, and some evidence of its existence in France predates the revolutionary era. But physicians were able to take full advantage of the opportunities afforded by the revolutionary climate, and vastly changed and expanded the scope of the French hospital system.

The new emphasis was on the hospital as a teaching institution, as a center for investigation, and on treatment based on clinical practice. A protocol of treatment based on experience and experimentation would replace the venerable unchallenged texts of bygone authorities.

Disease was now to be viewed as specific; old concepts of humoural balance were discarded. A new anatomical pathology was the replacement. The old emphasis on discussion of symptoms, external examination, and medical history, were replaced by an emphasis on what was going on inside the patient's body. The furtherance of medical knowledge for this purpose was enhanced by two factors. One was the presence of large numbers of human subjects to observe in the wards of the hospitals. The other was the invention of a fundamental diagnostic tool by a French physician named Laennee, of the stethescope in 1819. His rigid one–ear listening device, although eminently successful, was eventually replaced by a two–eared flexible listening tube, invented by the American physician, George Cammann, in 1852, thereby providing the modernized stethescope.

Listening to actual internal body sounds was far more objective than listening to a patient described set of symptoms. But this development carried with it the unfortunate side effect of weakening the personal relationship that dialogue had previously created between physician and patient. Over time the patient would be viewed less as a person, more as a body upon which to perform tests and then attempt corrective procedures based on the results of those tests.

The French approach would dominate the early nineteenth century, but its influence would also stimulate developments in other countries. The English made some notable additions to medical knowledge. Thomas Hodgkins, who introduced the French stethescope in London, discovered the disease named after him, Hodgkin's Disease. Thomas Addison discovered Addison's Disease, the Irishman, Robert Graves, discovered Grave's Disease (hyperthyroidism). Henry Gray first published *Gray's Anatomy* in 1858. In various edited forms it still exists.

In America there is little to celebrate medically in the nineteenth century. A few American physicians made the pilgrimage to France and returned to practice French style medicine. Commercialism and egalitarianism combined to provide a barren soil in which significant advances could take root. The American Medical Association was founded in 1847, but remained of little influence during its century of inception. Perhaps the most singular event in America concerned Andrew Carnegie's numerous trips to his native Scotland during the latter nineteenth century, where, most likely, he became aware of the advanced medical training being provided at Edinburgh. This would become of immense significance in the early twentieth century, when Carnegie and Rockefeller millions would redefine the scope of American medicine.

Whereas nineteenth century France dominated the medical scene from a clinical perspective, nineteenth century German states pursued a histological perspective. Whereas the French stethescope provided a basic diagnostic tool needed for the clinical approach, the Germans perfected the microscope and slide preparation during the course of the century. And it was not the hospital, but rather the university, that would become the institutional backbone of the German system and also as a symbol of rising German nationalism.

Research and scholarship were to be highly revered, and were substantially financed by government. The modern research university traces its origins to the German states, wherein significant individuals made their mark on medical advance. The list includes Justus von Leibig in chemistry and rudimentary biochemistry, and Karl Ernst von Baer in embryology. Karl Ludwig, Director of the influential Physiological Institute of Leipzig, advanced the position that medicine must be quantitative, analytical, and chemical. Rudolph Virchow established cell theory. He believed that new cells were created by the division of preexisting cells. Disease is the product of cells gone awry and then perpetuating their defect through further division.

Germ Theory

Undeniably, the greatest achievement of the nineteenth century was the discovery that certain diseases and infections were caused by minute living organisms. This theory had been subject to speculation for over two thousand years, but required the conclusive validation provided by the experiments of Louis Pasteur. Proving that the souring of milk and the fermenting of wine were not chemical, but rather bacterial processes, Pasteur was able to discover bacteria that ultimately led to cures for anthrax, chicken cholera, and rabies. Disease was caused in the body when it was invaded by microorganisms, and these could be identified. Known as germ theory, Pasteur's ideas were advanced by Joseph Lister in introducing antiseptic practices in the conduct of surgery, and by Alexander Gordon and others, in the practice of midwifery. Infection from surgery and deaths associated with childbirth dropped dramatically (see below).

Germ theory held that disease was the result of external forces invading the body. But a contemporary of Pasteur's, Claude Bernard, who had made numerous contributions to the field of medicine, proposed that this was not the entire story. He observed that not everyone who came in contact with the same disease actually contracted it. Obviously, simply coming into contact with a germ was not in itself disease causing. Bernard suggested that it was the "terrain," or, the environment with which the germ interacted, that actually made the difference. Today, we refer to the strengthening of the immune system –the terrain—as a propitious way to ward off disease. In later life Pasteur is reputed to have agreed that it was not the germ, but the condition of the host to resist the germ, that made all the difference. But by that time germ theory was totally enmeshed in the medical mind.

Pasteur's approach is essentially allopathic medicine; it focuses on treating disease by killing the invading organism (pathogen). The resultant carnage is oftentimes both indiscriminant and extensive. Bernard's approach is essentially naturopathic. Utilize natural substances to create maximum health. The premise is that the body would thereby be able to ward off the invading pathogens. Hohenheim's chemical medicine and Pasteur's germ theory did much to shape the modern course of medicine.

Pharmacology, as a distinct specialty, is a product of the nineteenth century. Numerous drugs were identified and isolated from their natural sources during the early nineteenth century. The dominant figures in this regard include the Frenchmen, Francois Magendie and Pierre Pelletier. Once isolated, chemical substances could be enhanced by concentration and also administered in specific dosages. Quinine, codeine, morphine, and cocaine, and at least another dozen lesser well known drugs, were soon in everyday use.

The French clinical approach emphasized pathology; the German laboratory approach emphasized physiology and pharmacology. The significance of Claude Bernard is that he used physiology to bridge the approaches, and made physiology the scientific basis for medicine. But scientific medicine required scientific quantitative devices, and these were to mushroom during the nineteenth century. In addition to the stethescope, and the earlier thermometer, a notable achievement was the invention of a device for measuring blood pressure, the sphygmomanometer.

Standards were set for what constituted a normal body temperature and normal blood pressure. Deviation from the norm indicated the presence of specific diseases. During the course of the century some chemical tests were devised to help determine the presence of certain diseases. Urinalysis provided useful information on body chemistry that indicated disease.

Pertaining to the field of surgery the nineteenth century opened with but a handful of standard operations. These generally consisted of amputations due to accident or disease (with a majority of patients dying from infection), repairing of tissue damaged by gunshot wounds generally resulting from incessant European warfare, and removal of cysts and tumors. Little of this could be termed intricate, nor could it have been. Speed of the procedure was of the essence, in that anesthetics were in the future.

Still, whenever a newly developed surgical procedure appeared, it became the fad, with the twentieth century well represented. An ovariotomy was first performed in the United States in 1809, and hundreds more immediately followed accompanied by a high mortality rate. Hysterectomies, mastectomies, and clitoridectomies were frequently performed nineteenth century operations, often with little or no medical basis.

Alcohol, opium, and mandrake root were given to dull the pain, but they were used sparingly due to the dangers their use contained. Ether was successfully used in the United States in the early 1840's by Thomas Morton, at Massachusetts General Hospital, and its use spread to Europe within a few years. Ether was both irritating to the membranes and nauseating, and although its use would continue into the twentieth century, chloroform soon replaced it. Ironically, chloroform had been around since the 1830's, but pain management did not seem to be a priority at the time. The Scot, James Young Simpson, demonstrated the use of chloroform at Edinburgh in 1847. Equally insensitive was the fact that the pain numbing effects of nitrous oxide (laughing gas) were well known as of

1800, but the substance was at the time only used for its entertainment value.

Ether and chloroform were general anesthetics possessed of possible serious side effects. Hence, their sparing use for all but the most invasive surgical procedures, while the search for something else continued. What was desired was a local anesthetic to be used for minor and localized surgical procedures. Cocaine was isolated from coca leaves in 1859 and was quickly proven to be an effective local anesthetic.

Another major impediment to successful surgery was the constantly present specter of infection. An estimated half of all patients undergoing routine surgeries died from infections. Childbirth fever was rampant, particularly in hospitals—much less so in home deliveries attended by midwives. It seemed that hospitals were places where sick people went to contract fatal disease. Physicians who suggested that unsanitary conditions and bacteria were responsible, were scoffed at by their less enlightened colleagues.

Early enlightened practitioners included the Scot, Alexander Gordon, the American, Oliver Wendell Holmes, and the Austrian, Ignaz Semmelweis. But it was Joseph Lister who came up with a preventative—carbolic acid. Bath the wound with carbolic acid, spray the operating room with carbolic acid, continually redress the wound with carbolic acid, and ipso facto, a vastly significant reduction in infections. Lister's discovery was welcomed with ridicule by his profession. Surgical procedures during the Franco–Prussian War, performed by surgeons on both sides who ignored Lister's findings, approximated a seventy five percent mortality rate. This necessitated some radical rethinking and Lister's carbolic acid became more widely used.

But there were still some problems. Surgeons still operated with bare hands and rarely scrubbed. The American, William Halsted, invented rubber gloves—an advance—although his was a different purpose. It seemed that constant exposure to carbolic acid was very irritating to the skin. The gloves were to prevent exposure to carbolic acid, but the unintended effect was a more sterile environment for surgical procedures.

The Prussian, Ernst von Bergmann, introduced steam sterilization of surgical instruments. The Pole, Johannes von Mikulicz–Radecki, introduced the surgical mask. Last to come was the gradually adoption of the use of the surgical gown (rather than street clothes), and the sanitizing and restricting of the operating area (generally a public audience was in open attendance at many surgeries). As a consequence, anesthetics and antiseptics, coupled with basic common sense sanitation, radically changed the success rate of surgery. The end of the nineteenth century witnessed far safer procedures than at its opening.

Medical Specialization

The scientific age had ushered in the scientific method. which called for discovery and validation of scientific principles in part by reducing them to their most fundamental components. The mid eighteenth century had brought the introduction of the factory system, replete with division of labor and specialization of task. As medical knowledge itself became increasingly specific, the generalist found it increasingly difficult to keep pace. In all walks of life, in all endeavors, specialization and differentiation were becoming the norm. It should not be surprising, then, that medical specialties began to appear. The result was significant advance in medical knowledge, but as we shall see in the next chapter, there was a price to be paid in turf battles and organizational disputes.

In England, and especially in the United States, obstetrics as a specialty was played down. This was a woman's matter to be handled by women. In the rest of Europe the formal upgrading of midwifery and its training was being witnessed. But pediatrics as a specialty marks its beginnings in the mid eighteenth century and a hospital devoted to the care of children was established in England in 1850. An orthopedic hospital had been established during the preceding decade. Orthopedics would developed into a solid specialty during the World War I era, undoubtedly encouraged by the carnage then present.

Specialties for ears, teeth, and throat developed during the nineteenth century, undoubtedly aided by the invention of specialized diagnostic instruments. The ophthalmoscope (1851) and the ophthalmometer (1852) were invented by Heimholz, while the laryngoscope (1855) was invented by Manuel Garcia. Specialties would continue to develop as specialized instruments and procedures were developed, and as the century wore on, hospitals were founded devoted to specific conditions. Skin, nervous disorders, colon and rectal, chest , urology, and cancer, all made it to the specialty list by century's end. Few specialists existed in the United States. The widely disseminated American population precluded all but the dense eastern seaboard from such development.

By 1900 medical specialization was well established, but there did exist an ongoing battle over status. Medical generalists regarded themselves as universal experts and the specialist as being narrow in perspective, and therefore incomplete in his medical knowledge. Specialization would make it impossible for the medical profession to achieve the unified organization it so much desired.

Public Health Issues

On the downside the nineteenth century had witnessed the growth of industrialization and concomitant urbanization. The concentration of people in crowded conditions predated adequate public health concerns. Not only were concentrated masses of people a potential health issue in itself, but inadequate sewerage systems, polluted water supplies, foul air in factory towns, and toxic substances emanating from manufacturing processes, all contributed to horrible living conditions.

These new urbanites were following the jobs. The jobs were in cities and factory operators at the time paid scant attention to health, safety, and environmental issues. Charles Dickens described the squalor in nineteenth century industrial England. His description could apply to the industrial centers of America as well. And it was those same conditions that inspired Karl Marx, as he peered from his smoke stained window in 1840's England.

Epidemics repeatedly slammed through the new industrial centers of the western world. Abbreviated lives were lived in squalid conditions. The sheer magnitude of the problem forced relatively indifferent governments to enter the public health arena. The rate at which people were dying, and their general lack of vigor, was viewed as a serious detriment to the continuance of the state. The emergence of public health organizations will be dealt with in the next chapter.

Europe certainly had more than its share of indigenous diseases, but it exacerbated its condition due to its geographical expansion. History already offered many examples of the spread of disease through contact with other civilizations, but generally, resultant medical disasters were relatively short lived.. Europe spread its conquering armies and agents over the globe with every intention of permanent occupation. Local diseases presented themselves as a very serious obstacle to the success of world domination. In fact, the very survival of imperialism itself depended on the ability to control local disease.

Europe had little experience with malaria before its era of expansionism except for some low lying regions in Italy. But malaria was spread around the world by sailing ship, and periodically ravaged the world. Mercifully, it generally contained itself along coastal regions, but even reached the northeastern portions of the United States. What caused malaria was at first unknown. Finally, in 1897, the Englishman, Ronald Ross, proved that the disease was transmitted by mosquitoes. The Italian, Giovanni Grassi, was able to identify which species of mosquito, as well as the various stages of its life cycle. A parasite residing in the stomachs of a particular mosquito was the culprit. No cure for the disease has been discovered, but considerable success at prevention was achieved. Mosquito control, chemically treating stagnant ponds, netting, window screens, and eventually DDT, had quite effectively controlled the disease by the end of World War II. But then two problems arose. The mosquitoes mutated, developing an immunity to DDT, and then DDT itself was proven to constitute an environmental hazard and discontinued. Worldwide, millions still die annually from the disease.

Yellow fever is also transmitted by a species of mosquito. This fact was suspected by the Cuban, Carlos Finlay, in 1881, and the Italian, Guiseppi Sanarelli, isolated the bacteria in 1897. Following the Spanish–American War, the Reed Commission, under the auspices of the United States Army, reconfirmed these findings and battled the disease in the same manner as malaria. The endeavor made possible the building of the Panama Canal. The eradication programs worked. A vaccine was formulated in 1937 but yellow fever remains a world disease.

A myriad of other tropical diseases were isolated. Most medical advances were the work of various religious missionaries or private philanthropic organizations such as the International Health Board, funded by the Rockefeller Foundation. Few cures resulted, but many causes were discovered. To the present day the major weapons against tropical disease are largely public health related. Since most countries suffering the most from tropical diseases are among the poorest nations on the planet, market driven pharmaceutical companies do not give tropical disease a high priority.

Chemical Medicine

Scientific reductionism was burrowing in on the secrets of the human body. Arteries, veins, and ducts were known due to the work of earlier dissectors. And by the mid nineteenth century internal bodily secretions that moved about in a ductless environment, yet were essential to human life, had been discovered. These ductless moving substances were given the name "hormones" in 1905. The role of the thyroid in metabolism regulation, and the significance of iodine in the process, had been discovered in 1895. The adrenal and its function as a blood pressure regulator soon followed. Then came the pituitary that regulated growth and the hypothalamus, as the chemical control center. Finally, in 1922, the role of the pancreas in blood sugar regulation and the function of insulin became known. Male and female hormones became known in the 1930's, and this eventually led to the development of oral contraceptives in 1959.

The modern chemical approach to medicine was pioneered by Paul Ehrlich. His work led to the discovery that a chemical compound, salvarsan, was effective against syphilis. Improved versions evolved into the modern day drug of choice, neoarsphenamine. Another early leader in chemotherapy was Gerhard Domagk, research director for a German chemical dye company. He discovered that a certain dye, prontosil red, was effective against streptococcal infections. Scientists at the Pasteur Institute isolated the chemical responsible, sulphonamide (the chemical had been known for several decades, but not its use). Various other sulpha drugs were soon developed that were effective against a variety of diseases. Sulpha drugs operate by preventing the reproduction of invading bacteria, giving the body time to marshal its defenses. A negative for the treatment was that streptococci mutate and develop resistance.

The objective then became one of tinkering with compounds, adding and subtracting ingredients, to find a more effective drug, or one with less side effects. Practically every chemical treatment discovered split into numerous variations, partly due to commercial competition, partly due to refined information, and in time, partly to deal with resistant mutations in the pathogen itself.

Folk medicine had long utilized mold as a dressing for wounds. The mold (fungi) killed other pathogens; the term for this is bacterial antagonism. Eventually substances that performed this way were called antibiotics. Penicillin was observed and suspected as to its efficacy in the late 1920's by Alexander Fleming. But it was not until the late 1930's when a team of Oxford University researchers successfully isolated penicillin in a form in which it could be used. Its commercial development took place in the United States due to the advent of war in Europe. Widely used, sometimes carelessly or too generously ever since, penicillin was discovered to diminish in its effect through continued use. Although one of the safest of all antibiotics, increasingly it is being replaced by harsher antibiotics. And some pathogens are naturally resistant to penicillin. Broad spectrum antibiotics were developed in the 1950's.

Robert Koch refined the micro organic process. Using solid cultures grown in a special dish designed by Richard Petri (the Petri dish), he was able to microscopically view organism without distortion. And whereas Pasteur had reproduced diseases in animals and then sought out the cause, the result was artificially induced disease. Cholera is a human disease; the discovery of chicken cholera is of no direct human consequence. Koch identified the tuberculosis bacillus and the cholera bacillus. His students went on to identify the organisms responsible for diptheria, typhoid, tetanus, pneumonia, gonorrhea, and leprosy.

Identifying a cause does not affect a cure. The German, Emil Gehring, and his Japanese colleague, Shibasaburo Kitasato developed a serum anti-toxin. Researchers at the Koch Institute discovered how to use serum of an immune animal to protect against the disease, and serum anti toxin therapy soon followed. Two Frenchmen at the Pasteur Institute, Albert Calmette and Jean Marie Guerin, discovered a substantive treatment for tuberculosis in the 1920's.

Viral infections are fluid, much less specific, and cannot be attacked with antibiotics. Vaccines discovered in th 1950's and 1960's were effective against some, notably polio, mumps, and measles. Chemical drugs have had some success against herpes related viruses. The influenza virus continually mutates. There has been a price paid for the chemical revolution. A case in point was the sleeping pill, thalidomide, a drug that caused massive birth defects.

Some diseases, it was discovered, were caused, not by invading agents, but by the lack of some vital substance in the body. The list of diseases included pellagra, beriberi, rickets, scurvy, and pernicious anemia. In 1912 Casimir Funk isolated the substance preventing beriberi, and called it a vitamine. During the 1920's and early 1930's basic vitamins had been discovered. The research, however, had uncovered a serious problem. Essential substances were being destroyed or discarded as part of food processing, and issues of "junk food" emerged as a modern concern.

Another avenue of attack is found in the field of immunology. Certain pathogens, notably viruses, did not respond to antibiotics and therefore demanded a different approach. Research on how the body defends itself was taking place parallel to the advances in chemical medicine. Antibodies were discovered and investigated. The role of white blood cells in immune activity was becoming known. Immunizing the body against certain pathogens was making progress. (This subject will be dealt with in greater detail in the discussion on public health.)

Pharmacology had become an integral part of medical research. It was discovered in nerve research that stimulation caused the secretion of various naturally occurring chemical agents that caused the actions of muscles and organs. Once these chemicals were isolated, other chemicals could then be developed to enhance or retard their action. Additionally, it was discovered that chemical substances could be used to control brain function. This would lead to Harvard based research on lysergic acid diethylamide, popularly known as LSD. Essentially, psychotropic drugs inhibit neurotransmitter functioning. Dopamine, for instance, somewhat inhibits the symptoms of Parkinson's disease. Psychopharmacological drugs are now being dispensed like candy.

One of the most dreaded words of the modern era is the word "cancer," a disease that has persisted since ancient times, although not with such intensity as now. In 1867 Wilhelm Waldeyer suggested that cancer cells originated from normal cells. A few decades later it was discovered that certain substances cause cancers to develop. This led to the belief that chemical solutions could be found. But specific chemicals for specific cancer cells were not found. Instead, a chemical shotgun approach has been used that fails to distinguish between cancer cells and healthy cells, a condition equally true for radiation treatment. Side effects can be catastrophic. Surgical procedures can physically remove many cancerous organs or malignant tumors, but do not address the causes. Systemic cancers are beyond the scope of surgical skills.

Chemical success with leukemia has been noteworthy. But as yet no cure for cancer has been discovered. Yet some cancer victims do survive. The paradigm of science and of pharmacology has rendered it difficult for medical researchers to seek less than exotic solutions. Since we know the types of substances or behaviors that cause cancer, why cannot the same approach toward cancer that was used toward malaria be utilized? Billions are spent each year on cancer research alone, but scant resources are devoted to inexpensive preventive strategies.

Twentieth Century Killers

There has been notable success in cancer detection, and early detection is a major factor in cancer survival, with the advent of MRI's and CATscans. Monoclonal antibody treatment, if conjoined with radioactive isotopes, can seek out, identify, and destroy specific cancer cells while ignoring healthy cells. The procedure shows considerable promise, and avoids many of the side effects of standard allopathic cancer treatment, but currently it is astronomically expensive.

Immunology, as a possible preventive, has received minimal support. News releases periodically focus on a possible cancer vaccine, or someone hypes a miracle cure. Cancer research is big business, responsible for many lifetime careers. The research techniques involved are very time consuming and very expensive. Yet while cancer research goes on the market continues to be flooded with known carcinogenic products. Society has moved to the concept of "acceptable risk," gambling on health for commercial motives. The public continues to use or ingest products that are proven harmful, yet only one such product has been singled out for attack—tobacco.

Cancer is not the only major twentieth century killer. Cardiovascular disease is a twentieth century disease. Diagnosis was made possible by the invention of the electrocardiograph in 1903, and the ability to accurately interpret its information by the 1920's. Hypertension and arteriosclerosis were identified as leading precursors of myocardial infraction (heart attack). Exotic invasive measures, open heart surgeries, were introduced during the 1960's. Initially marginal in their success rates, these procedures soon became routine, and were a boon to many people who had no other remaining options. Beta blockers for angina and reduction of blood pressure, blood thinners, clot dissolvers, have all been useful tools.

Defibrillators and pace makers regulate heart rhythm, sometimes saving lives and often improving the quality of life. An understanding of the role of cholesterol and subsequent adjustment of life style are major preventive measures to lessen the risk of heart disease. Prevention has an absolute proven effect on reducing the risk of heart attack.

Inherited Disease

It has long been suspected that certain diseases were of an hereditary nature, gout, for instance. Scientific evidence supporting this belief was obtained by work with sickle cell anemia in the 1900's and Down's syndrome in the 1950's. In 1953 Francis Crick and James Watson discovered the double helix DNA chain. (DNA had been discovered in the 1920's but its role was not correctly understood.) By the 1980's the genetic code contained within the DNA could be distinguished chemically. It then became possible to eventually identify and determine the role of each individual gene. This led to the human genome project. Powerful computers accelerated the completion of its goal—to map the entire human genetic code.

The fallout from this project has already been stupendous, leading to further understanding of issues other than medical, such as early human migration patterns. In time it will be possible to identify a potentially defective gene, repair it, and prevent that particular disease from surfacing fifty years later. Some medical scientists are predicting success by around 2020; others believe it could take a hundred years. But many ethicists are raising serious questions.

The cloning of a sheep in Scotland, and the decision made in the United Kingdom early in 2001 to proceed with a human cloning project, raise disturbing issues. Human cloning is currently banned in the United States, but the prospects of a genetically engineered "master race," or of humans bred to fulfill specific functions, will certainly not be lost on the demented of the world. If history is any indication, humanity has been rather consistent in using scientific advances for destructive ends. Life is an adventure; to know in advance its end might well destroy the plot. Knowledge of one's genetic structure could led to employment discrimination, the "defective gene" defense in legal proceedings (how would it differ from the insanity plea?), programming for one's offspring, serious challenges to privacy issues, in effect, *Brave New World*.

But it now appears that as formidable as the human genome project has been, there is another even more formidable challenge ahead. It seems that each of the roughly 40,000 genes in the human body contain the same genetic letters. The trick lies in their sequencing. The next step is to identify all of the proteins in the body, and it has been suggested that there might be a million of them. Science is already getting a handle on how to proceed. The end result will have staggering consequences. So the name of the new game is proteome.

If properly used, the knowledge to be acquired should be of immense benefit to humankind. This knowledge, if conjoined with advances currently being made in the field of energy medicine, offer tremendous potential for the future.

Issues of Immunity

The late twentieth century raised issues concerning immunity. There are two basic types of immunity: natural and acquired. Acquired immunity can be active, that is, the body makes what it needs, or passive, the immunity is received from outside the body. The big concern involves acquired passive immunity.

Studies with blood and its eventual typing, as well as early errors in attempted transfusions, led to the discovery that there were natural antibodies in humans, that under the proper circumstances they cloned themselves to meet demand, and eventually, that thymus, or T cells, were needed to make the process work. The body possesses a very complex process whereby it determines what is not of its own "self," and it is designed to destroy whatever it does not recognize.

AIDS, or Acquired Immuno–Deficiency Syndrome, is caused by a virus that attacks white blood cells and shuts down the process by which the natural immune system is maintained. The virus itself has been named the Human Immuno–Deficiency Virus, or, HIV. Infectious diseases are only treatable by soliciting the aid of the body's natural immune system. If no natural immune system is present, then there can be no successful treatment and the invading pathogens would win. People with AIDS are at enormous risk As yet, there is no cure for AIDS. There are a variety of drug cocktails that have been proven successful in suppressing the virus that causes AIDS. There are a number of celebrities who have contracted the HIV, who have been able to suppress the manifestation of AIDS.

Advances in Surgery

Significant advances occurred in twentieth century surgery. Previously mentioned nineteenth century advances in anesthetics and sterilization had clearly rendered surgery less risky and more successful, but the surgeon continued to remain low on the medical status totem pole. To attain the status it was beginning to deserve, some positive public relations had to occur. It came from two sources.

First, in the nineteenth century, the writings and flamboyant behavior of Theodor Billroth, provided considerable popularization of surgery. Billroth was both brilliant and careless. The two traits combined to produce many innovative surgical techniques, and Billroth was widely emulated. By the early twentieth century surgeries were becoming routine, fashionable, and occasionally faddish.

Brain tumors were successfully removed beginning around the opening of the twentieth century. The mortality rate for this procedure dropped appreciably over the course of the century. The leading pioneer American neurosurgeon was Harvey Cushing.

The appendectomy was the most popular operation of the 1930's. Any form of stomach cramp or pain was immediate grounds for surgery. In its place the operation is a relatively risk free life saving procedure. In the 1930's and 1940's the operation of choice was the tonsillectomy. All that was required was a sore throat. Might as well take out the adenoids at the same time. The role of the glands in the body's immune system was ignored. Neither surgery is performed today with the same frequency. And then the hysterectomy, the most performed unnecessary operation of the twentieth century. All that was necessary to be a candidate for this procedure was to be menopausal or a little irregular. The radical mastectomy ran a close second. Any lump or bump made a person a candidate. By the 1970's. after eighty years performing this procedure, the medical profession came to the conclusion that, in most cases less invasive surgery was just as effective. The lock step mentality of the medical establishment can often be a major detriment to the well being of the patients it serves.

What did the most to establish the efficacy of surgery in the public mind was the creation of a surgical hospital in Rochester, Minnesota. Founded by the Mayo brothers, both surgeons, the hospital utilized numerous monitoring and testing procedures, and successfully routinized many surgical procedures. The safeguards employed at the Mayo Clinic produced a high success rate, instilled a public confidence, and established a Mayo surgery as a status symbol

New and exotic surgical procedures make headlines, and surgeons today enjoy high status in the medical profession. But although modern surgery clearly saves lives, improves the quality of life, or simply extends life for a time, surgery is not the entire answer. It is not a cure for certain chronic conditions such as cancer. Cutting away a cancerous tumor does not effect a cure for cancer; yet it may prolong life, and in conjunction with other healing modalities, achieve some success.

But in certain areas surgery has achieved remarkable success. The first angiocardiogram was performed in 1931, soon followed by catherization, and eventually, in 1964, the first angioplasty. Anastomosis (the sewing together of veins or arteries) was established in 1910, and would eventually make possible more invasive heart procedures, notably transplants. At first surgeons bought time in performing their procedures by lowering the body temperature (hypothermia) to reduce the heart beat. Over time various surgical repair procedures were perfected. In 1953 a heart lung machine was successfully used , making possible longer and more exotic heart surgeries than were possible in the past. By the 1950's, valve replacement procedures, necessitating open heart surgery , became common. The pacemaker appeared in 1959, and in 1967 the first bypass operation was performed.

Advances in reconstructive, or plastic, surgery, would pave the way for heart transplants. First came skin and cornea transplants. But experimentation with organ transplants (in animals) surfaced a new challenge—rejection. The body's natural defense mechanism, its immune system, would literally fight to the death to kill any foreign substance. Before organ transplants could successfully take place, immunosuppressant drugs had to be developed.

Cyclosporine, in the late 1970's, made this possible. It was initially used to conjunction with kidney transplants. Kidney transplant posed less challenge. The kidney can be tissue typed, and there was usually a spare, and in a worse case scenario, there was always dialysis. The only real issue was one of compatibility. The first successful kidney transplant occurred in Boston in 1954. It was followed by a lung transplant and a liver transplant in 1963. Christiaan Bernard performed the world's first heart transplant in South Africa in 1967. A hundred more such operations occurred around the world during the following year. The surgical procedures for these transplants were perfected, but most patients soon died. Note that they preceded the introduction of cyclosporine. The cause of surgical progress was dearly paid for by early transplant "victims." Is such also the case with current artificial heart recipients?

Severed limbs were reattached as of 1962; an artificial hip replacement occurred in 1972. A reattached severed penis made world headlines in 1993. Synthetic and natural body replacements are becoming commonplace. As a consequence, the issue of organs for sale, using the organs of executed individuals, who on an organ waiting list has priority, and sundry other issues, raise thorny questions for medical ethicists.

If ethical problems exist over organ transplant, and they do, the issue compounds itself in the area of human reproduction. Medical science has made some major advances in the area of fertility. In vitro fertilization entered the scene in 1969, with a ten percent success rate. Artificial insemination soon followed. These procedures were a boon to some infertile couples, but presented a host of issues outside of the field of medicine. With the advent of surrogate mothers and sperm donor fathers, issues of paternity and maternity are no longer clearly delineated.

Radiation

Other medical procedures were developed during the course of the twentieth century. In 1895 Karl Rontgen discovered x ray. The following year it was being used to peer into the human body, and proved to be an excellent diagnostic tool. The dangers of over exposure to x ray were already noted in 1902. At the end of 1898 the Curie's discovered radium. Since its rays burned, could they not be directed toward diseased cells? By the opening of the twentieth century radiation treatment for cancer was a reality

X ray and radiation became the rage. Machines to view the foot inside a shoe were in most shoe stores until the 1940's. No heed was paid to duration or frequency of exposure. The effects and the dangers of radiation were ignored until after the exploding of the atomic bomb. Even then the federal government, in its civilian defense films, claimed one could only contract radiation sickness through an unprotected open wound or by keeping one's mouth open. Radiation particles, the American public was told, bounced off the skin. Troops maneuvered under atomic blasts so the government could determine how much radiation they could withstand. And this was after the events at Hiroshima and Nagasaki. The general public was advised to "duck and cover," to protect them from atomic blasts. Meanwhile the government was expending vast sums burrowing underground to provide safe havens of "duck and cover" for itself. Check the video *Atomic Café.*

Light Amplification by Stimulated Emission of Radiation (LASER) was originally theorized by Einstein and became a most useful surgical tool. Laser surgery is clean, neat, and practically bloodless. It is computer controlled and therefore excellent for minute, precise cuts. It is widely used in corneal operations, microscopic surgeries, and a variety of cosmetic procedures.

Constantly improved microscopes provided the equipment that led to further advances in medical science. Electron microscopes first appeared in the 1930's. By the 1970's there were scanning electron microscopes. A notable diagnostic breakthrough occurred when the Scot, Ian Donald, used Sound Navigation and Ranging (SONAR) on human tissue to diagnose tumors. Later it was used to view fetal development. Sound diagnosis was in use by the late 1950's and apparently carried with it no known side effects. Another diagnostic tool was the infra–red ray, used to scan the human body for "hot spots," which generally indicated a diseased area.

In 1967 Godfrey Hounsfeld developed Computerized Axial Tomography. In this process a series of fine x rays scan the body and are processed into a 3D image by computer. Hence the term CAT–Scan. This eventually led to Magnetic Resonance Imaging (MRI). A three dimensional image is obtained by resonating the body's hydrogen atoms magnetically, and then processing the data obtained by computer. A significant advantage of this tool lies in the fact that it utilizes no radiation.. Another related diagnostic tool is Positive Emission Transaxial Tomography (PETT). This process scans the brain with injected radioactive glucose.

Medicine has made significant strides over the centuries. Modern scientific medicine is saving the lives of many people who would have died just a few decades ago. But as it becomes increasingly complex, the opportunity for error increases. Iatrogenically induced illness, or even death, is a growing, very real threat that the medical establishment needs to address very seriously. Allopathic medicine is complex; there is a price to be paid for success. The medical profession is praised and the medical profession is condemned.

The goal of this book is to neither praise nor condemn. It is simply to enable readers to ask intelligent questions of their health care professionals, and to make fully informed decisions concerning their medical care. And this is the direction of the remaining chapters.

Chapter Summary

- Modern medicine developed during a time of revolutionary change. This eased and accelerated its ascendancy.
- France provided early leadership, emphasizing hospitals as teaching institutions, and developing new diagnostic instruments. The French approach was clinical; the German approach was histological.

- A monumental event of the nineteenth century was the development of germ theory, which held that disease is caused by invading microorganisms. Major figures involved are Pasteur and Lister.
- Bernard countered with terrain theory, which held that disease could not take hold in a healthy environment—a strong immune system.
- Pasteur's approach is essentially allopathic medicine, especially when combined with Hohenheim's chemical medicine.
- Early nineteenth surgery was characterized by high mortality rates. Infection was the leading culprit. Since anesthetics were in the future, speed was the most prized skill in a surgeon.
- By mid century ether and chloroform were used as general anesthetics; cocaine was a local anesthetic.
- By 1900 carbolic acid, surgical gloves and masks, and sterile fields, massively reduced death by infection.
- Medical specialization developed during the course of the nineteenth century.
- Public health became a major concern in the nineteenth century as urban epidemics were rampant. This was partly due to crowded unsanitary urban conditions and partly due to contact with tropical diseases brought on by expansionism.
- The early twentieth century witnessed advances in the identification and purposes of the body's glandular system.
- Chemical medicine was in the ascendancy throughout the twentieth century. Ehrlich pioneered the modern chemical approach. First came sulpha drugs, then penicillin, and eventually, broad spectrum antibiotics.
- The mid twentieth century witnessed the development of vaccines effective for a variety of diseases. Most notable was the polio vaccine.

- Widespread acceptance and use of chemical medicine has not come without a price. There have been disasters and there have been failures. Emphasis remains on finding the "magic bullet."
- Cancer and cardiovascular disease were the top killers of the twentieth century. The response has been exotic and highly invasive procedures, with varying degrees of success. Health and commercialism are in conflict.
- The discovery of DNA, the mapping of the human genetic code, and eventually, cloning, has led to massive ethical controversy.
- Surgery has enjoyed enormous technological advances during the latter third of the twentieth century. Surgical transplants, partially made possible by the development of immuno suppressant drugs, have become commonplace.
- X-ray was discovered at the opening of the twentieth century, and was originally used as a diagnostic tool. It quickly became radiation treatment for cancer.
- Major high tech developments by the end of the twentieth century include LASER in surgery, and SONAR. CAT-Scan, MRI, and PETT in diagnosis.

Chapter Three

Medical Practitioners

There are many different types of health practitioners. In this chapter we shall consider those types that require an extensive accredited graduate level educational program leading to a conferred medical degree, whose standardized requirements are established by the recognized professional medical organization of their specific craft.. Further, we will consider those graduates only who are required to complete an internship and/or residency program and successfully pass a state administered licensing examination as a condition for practicing their craft.

However, this is not a "one size fits all" definition. A number of medical programs clearly fit these criteria, and their graduates are licensed in all fifty states. But there are a couple of exceptions that I am including in this chapter that do not entirely fit the parameters of our discussion, mainly due to the role they are beginning to play on the contemporary medical scene: homeopathy and naturopathy. Some might argue, on solid grounds, that these modalities belong in a discussion of alternative medicine. But a growing number of mainstream health professionals are incorporating progressively more of their approaches in their practices, and it is for this reason that I choose to consider them here.

In researching the material for this chapter I was somewhat surprised to observe the amount of vitriolic pronouncements made by health professionals concerning various healing professions not their own. It is to be noted, however, that these came from individuals and not from professional organizations. Despite the movement toward greater acceptance and toleration in the healing arts, it appears that the ancient turf battles are not entirely resolved. It is not the intention of this work to join in the fray, but rather to define various healing professions according to their own stated positions.

Doctor of Medicine

M.D. Mainstream medicine in the United States is dominated by the medical doctor (M.D.), and is popularly referred to as "allopathic" medicine. The terms "allopathic medicine" or "allopathic physician" can have two very different meaning, one positive, and the other considerably less so. The conflict presented by the formally trained physician who follows a prescribed program of study, as opposed to a host of other types of healers, has been present for a very long time. One only need recall the struggle between "regulars" and "irregulars" in European history.

The term "allopathic" was coined by Samuel Hahnemann, founder of homeopathy, in referring to the very unscientific and often deadly practices of many of his medical peers. By "allopathic" Hahnemann was referring to bloodletting, purging, and the dispensing of harsh unproven drugs. In the modern era the term generally refers to that practice of medicine that primarily utilizes medicines, surgery, and other more intrusive measures. That meaning is further refined by the American Medical Association's definition of "modern scientifically based biomedicine." A portion of the alternative movement uses the term in its most derisive sense as "slash, burn, and poison" medicine, or in a more mellow sense, as a form of medicine that emphasizes exotic intrusive procedures rather than less invasive procedures. We are here referring to allopathic medicine according to the definition of the American Medical Association.

As was observed in Chapter Two, medical training at its best in early America was rather mediocre. America rejected anything European, anything that smattered of elitism, anything that impinged on individualism. Medicine, what there was of it, was practiced in a libertarian, laissez faire atmosphere. It is not at all surprising that many alternative healing systems were either founded in, or discovered a fertile ground in the United States.

Most early medical colleges were of questionable quality. None were in any way accredited. A would–be practitioner either graduated from a medical college, and then entered practice (occasionally after apprenticing for a time), apprenticed under a practicing physician, and then entered practice, without any formal course of study, or simply just starting practicing. It was a rather sorry state.

In reaction to this state of affairs, a young New York physician, Nathan Smith (1817–1904), in an effort to "elevate the standard of medical education in the United States," proposed the establishment of a national medical association. Through his efforts, in 1847, the American Medical Association was formed. The initial success of the organization was minimal. The climate of America was overwhelmingly laissez faire, and the political system of the era was in agreement. Both the climate and the politics would change with the accession of Theodore Roosevelt to the presidency at the opening of the twentieth century. The political progressivism of the Roosevelt era leaned toward regulation and control.

In 1901 the AMA took upon itself the task of inspecting and rating the nation's medical schools. It accepted and endorsed the recommendations of the Flexner Report (see Chapter Four), which called for a massive overhaul of American medical education. In 1912 the AMA's rating of medical schools was accepted as the accrediting standard by the Federation of State Medical Boards.

Over the next two decades the AMA's Council on Medical Education established standards for hospital internships (1914), adopted standards for specialty training (1923), and recognized medical specialty boards (1934). In 1942 the Council on Medical Education established the M.D. accrediting program, and exactly thirty years later residency accreditation was added. Finally, since 1997, the AMA has maintained the American Medical Accreditation Program (AMAP), an elaborate system of licensing, certification, performance, and continuing education requirements.

Quite clearly the AMA has succeeded in its goal of establishing rigorous requirements for the practice of medicine. Following graduation from college in a premed program emphasizing the sciences, the candidate enrolls in medical schools. Medical school is a four year program, the successful completion of which confers the M.D. degree. Medical school is followed by three years in internship/residency for general practice. Additional years of residency are required for Board Certified specialties. General Surgery, for example requires five years; surgical subspecialties could tack on an additional one to four years.

There are currently twenty–four specialty boards approved by the AMA. Completion of residency requirements and successful examinations in the area of specialty, results in the awarding of "Diplomat" in that board specialty. Diplomats have continuing education requirements and periodic renewal of certification. The vast majority of M.D.'s seek Diplomat status. With no delays or interruptions, the average general practitioner is ready to begin practice at about the age of thirty. Some specialties could delay commencing practice until the mid to late thirties.

Standards are rigorous. Medical training is quite lengthy and very expensive. Somehow, approximately 16,000 graduates make it through the program each year. The end result is a very expensive, highly technical and complex medical system, capable of delivering excellent health care.

Doctor of Osteopathy

D.O. Osteopathy finds its roots in the American heartland. Andrew Taylor Still (1828–1917) was the son of a Methodist preacher–doctor (a common combination on the American frontier). The young Still learned medicine from his father and briefly attended a medical college before enlisting in the Union Army during the Civil War. He worked as a surgeon during the war, and afterwards, began the practice of medicine. He apparently never completed his formal medical training, again, not uncommon at the time. Following the death of his three children from spinal meningitis, he became thoroughly disenchanted with the medical practices of his day.

Still's study produced three principles: that the body produces its own healing substances, that health is dependent on the structural integrity of the body, and that perverted structure is the fundamental cause of disease. Manipulation became a major part of his therapy, but unlike the slightly later chiropractic, not to the exclusion of other forms of medical treatment. His catharsis occurred when he reputedly cured a child of dysentery through spinal manipulation. Osteopathic spinal abnormalities are called "areas of somatic dysfunction." His principle belief was that the musculoskeletal system was a major factor in disease, and therefore a major avenue for therapy. He founded the first college of osteopathy at Kirksville, Missouri, in 1892, where he personally taught his theories of spinal manipulation as well as other therapies available at the time.

Osteopaths currently receive a full conventional medical training in addition to specialized osteopathic studies. Seven years of training are required to become a fully certified D.O. Osteopathy is part science, part art, and part belief. In conventional training osteopaths are akin to medical doctors, and are fully licensed in all fifty states to prescribe drugs, perform surgery, sign death certificates, etc. What sets osteopathy apart is not the science and not the art, but the belief.

There are five basic premises upon which osteopathy is based. One is that the human body is an integrated unit in which its structures and its functions cannot be separated. Two, the human body is a self healing, self regulating system. Three, for it to accomplish self healing and self regulating properly, there must be a free flow of blood and nerve impulses. Four, the musculoskeletal system plays a role in body health far beyond its obvious mechanical purposes. And five, the musculoskeletal system can house, contribute to, or maintain, the disease process, either at the symptomatic site or remote from it, and treatment is usually possible.

If any alteration in the structure of the body occurs, then the function of the body will be affected. The effects of the alteration occur through the nervous system—if it is acting abnormally. Osteopathic manipulation aims to restore proper function. Problems in the musculoskeletal system can lead to breathing problems, blood and lymphatic circulatory problems, and displaced organs which can lead to pathological conditions. The main pathway of body function is through the spinal cord, an evolutionary aberration resulting from a quadruped walking upright. The structural design of human beings is not ideally suited for the upright position, and when combined with gravity, place constant stress on the spine.

If problems exist in the spinal cord, nerve impulses will be somewhat altered, leading to misinformation. The misinformation can be compounded due to the "facilitated segment," that is, injured areas are easier to access than normal areas for the nervous system, and they attract and exaggerate even very minor impulses, thereby exacerbating the imbalanced condition.

In its purest form osteopathy comprises an holistic approach to healing, and is preventive medicine oriented. However, many osteopathic colleges today, as well as their graduates, emphasize conventional procedures that are indistinguishable from that of medical doctors. Should the patient desire osteopathic treatment, it would be best to determine whether the D.O. was a member of the Academy of Applied Osteopathy.

This organization and its members profess to keep alive the precepts of early osteopaths.

Membership in the AMA is open to students and graduates of "accredited allopathic or osteopathic medical schools," but such was not always the case. In 1953, John W. Cline, M.D., former president of the AMA, personally investigated the status of osteopathic training, and presented his findings to the AMA in what became known as the Cline Report. It indicated that "no fundamental differences exist between Medicine and Osteopathy." But in the following year a paper presented before the AMA opposed any cooperation between medicine and osteopathy, and the AMA subsequently voted against recognition and cooperation. In 1959 the AMA offered recognition in exchange for control over the accrediting of osteopathic educational institutions. The offer was refused.

For much of their history, osteopaths tended to regard themselves as second–class doctors, admiring the status that medical doctors were accorded. Some abandoned osteopathy and practiced strictly conventional medicine. Something of an identity crisis had developed within the osteopathic profession. But the number of osteopathic training institutions has been growing, and osteopathy is licensed in all fifty states. Since the Sixties, osteopaths have been accorded full physician status in the military. The profession is now turning out twice as many graduates than it did a decade ago—some 2000 annually.

Roughly sixty percent of all practicing osteopaths belong to their own professional organization. A little less than forty percent follow allopathic medicine and do their residencies in allopathic hospitals. While the AMA has opposed the opening of new osteopathic colleges, claiming oversupply, osteopaths claim they are filling a void in medical care. It seems that medical doctors overwhelmingly prefer specialties while osteopaths tend to prefer primary care practices, even though specialization is also an option for them as well. Some sixty percent of osteopaths are primary care physicians; medical doctors comprise ten percent. The HMO delivery system is attracted to the osteopathic approach due to its emphasis on prevention and low cost interventions such as manipulation. Osteopathy is generally a lower cost healing modality than is conventional medicine.

As a result, D.O.'s are beginning to assert their own identity. After decades of seeking recognition from the AMA (which they are eligible to join), that desire is no longer a pressing one. In the late Nineties an offer was made to osteopaths to send voting delegates to the AMA House of Delegates, but it was declined. Today, however, there is far more cooperation and professional respect among the various types of health care practitioners than existed just a couple of decades ago.

Doctor of Chiropractic

D.C. Chiropractic has endured a stormy existence. The classic texts of antiquity referenced spinal manipulation, the two most influential physicians of the day, Hippocrates and Galen, having used it. Spinal manipulation was part of Arab medicine, and returned as a part of folk medicine to Europe with the advent of Renaissance medicine.

The fierce egalitarian democracy of nineteenth century America resulted in a number of distinctively American healing movements, many of which are mentioned throughout this text. Both osteopathy and chiropractic emerged out of this culture. But well before osteopathy or chiropractic came into existence, a conventionally trained physician, J. Evan Riadore, wrote a paper published in London in 1842, entitled "A Treatise on irritation of the Spinal Nerves as the Source of Nervousness, Indigestion, Functional and Organical Derangement of the Principle Organs of the Body...." In 1835 Riadore had given a series of lectures on "nervous irritation and spinal affections." Inasmuch as Riadore had lectured and written extensively, it is highly probable that the founder of osteopathy, Andrew Still, and the founder of chiropractic, Daniel Palmer, were both aware of his seminal work. Riadore might well be the common antecedent of both medical movements.

Daniel David Palmer (1845–1913), a native Canadian, made his living as a magnetic healer prior to discovering chiropractic in 1895. In his own words Palmer claimed to have restored the hearing of the janitor in his building by "racking a vertebra" into its normal position. A short time later, Palmer discovered a heart patient with a displaced vertebra pressing against the nerves of the heart, adjusted it, and healed the heart condition. He went on to found the first chiropractic school, Palmer College, in Davenport, Iowa.

Chiropractic was originally based on the "one cause, one cure" theory; spinal subluxations were at the root of ninety–five percent of all disease. The initial theory held that a misaligned vertebra pressed on nerves interrupting the proper flow of nerve impulses, causing imbalances which caused disease. Early chiropractors would adjust the misaligned vertebra, remove the blockage, ease pain, and promote healing. While it is certainly true that many patients experienced immediate relief, the theory itself was false and often misstated.

Chiropractic discovered an immediate foe in the AMA. That organization had taken upon itself in 1849 the task to define what was proper or improper treatment, while it was still debating whether anesthetics in surgery served any useful purpose. Many early chiropractors were charged with practicing medicine without a license and spent time in jail, including Palmer himself. The AMA attempted to drive chiropractic out of existence by mandating that its members not cooperate with chiropractors, not send patients to chiropractors, and not receive patients from chiropractors.

In a protracted anti trust suit commencing in 1976, and finally concluding in 1990, *Wilk et al v AMA et al,* the AMA and its members were found to have participated in a conspiracy against chiropractic in violation of federal anti trust laws. By the time the courts reached this decision, the AMA had ceased its professional boycott of chiropractic. Relations with the chiropractic profession were seen to rest, in certain circumstances, on a scientific basis. The AMA recognized improvements in the practice of chiropractic, and chiropractic itself had moved away from its one cause, one cure premise.

The move away from the earlier simplistic approach had actually begun in the 1930's by the Belgian, Henri Gillet, with the formulation of his intervertebral motion theory. Early attempts to document the positive effects of chiropractic were made by Bartlett Palmer, son of the founder, but his techniques did not meet the rigors of modern scientific inquiry (nor did few others at the time). Yet the gulf between medicine and chiropractic had continued to widen in America. In Europe, on the other hand, medical doctors and chiropractors were jointly investigating and researching. Such activity was late in coming to America.

In the 1970's Chung Ha Suh conducted scientific research on spinal joint mechanics, and Marvin Luttges did work on spinal nerve roots. In both Canada and the United Kingdom joint studies by chiropractors and orthopedic surgeons to determine efficacy and parameters of chiropractic treatment had been undertaken. The RAND study in the United States (1992) acknowledged some positive effects deriving from spinal manipulation. (There is always a danger for adherents to a therapy claiming more than is within the scope of their treatment.) A number of studies in the Nineties have shown chiropractic to be effective in treating musculoskeletal conditions.

Chiropractic is a drug free, non intrusive, non surgical modality. A chiropractic examination emphasizes the interconnectedness of the human body. An effect (pain) in one part of the body may have its cause in a different location. Attention is increasingly being given to neuromuscular conditions and diagnosis, which has the added benefit of being scientifically based and therefore more acceptable to conventional medicine. Chiropractic considers the body holistically and attempts to treat accordingly. Modern responsible chiropractors know their limits and refer patients to medical doctors in a timely manner when conditions warrant.

Modern chiropractic makes use of some of the diagnostic equipment used by allopathic medicine, for example, MRI's.

The American Chiropractic Association has been the sole accrediting agency for chiropractic colleges since the 1970's. Chiropractic is a four year course of study, culminating in the degree of Doctor of Chiropractic. The profession is licensed in fifty states.

There is some overlapping between osteopathy and chiropractic. Both professions may make use of soft tissue massage, and a massage therapist might be part of the office team. Related also is the work performed by physical therapists, part of which involves mechanical manipulation. This could be done in conjunction with the treatment prescribed by osteopath, chiropractor, or orthopedic surgeon. And finally, an integrated part of orthodox medicine, physiotherapy, employs techniques usually associated with alternative medicine, notably hydrotherapy.

Doctor of Naturopathy

N.D., N.M.D. The subject of naturopathy is approached with some trepidation. A working definition is difficult in that the profession itself is not agreed. In this discussion we will consider what is termed "naturopathic medicine," and also what is termed "traditional naturopathy." The former is championed by the American Association of Naturopathic Physicians, while the latter is represented by the Coalition for Natural Health. But before addressing this volatile issue, let us first consider the historic background of the movement and its classical identifying characteristics.

The historic roots of natural healing obviously date back to ancient times when no other form of healing existed. But in a more modern sense it dates from the nineteenth century spa movement started in Germany, and a host of populist health movements in America at the same time. First, let us consider the German story.

The movement begins with Vincenz Priessnitz, a shepard, who noticed that injured animals tended to seek out mountain streams and stand in them. From this Priessnitz posited that cold water healed. And from this inauspicious beginning there soon followed a network of health spas, located at the sites of natural springs. Hydrotherapy, or, the "water cure" became a national movement, to which was added other natural therapies: massage, exercise, herbs, and nutrition. To the present day spas are a part of German culture.

Meanwhile frontier America, with its romanticizing of the virtues of agrarian life, and a spirit of egalitarianism that somehow translated into an anti–intellectualism that lasts to the present day, was well entrenched in the natural way. After all, Thomas Jefferson had written that the most virtuous of people were the farmers. And various religious groups, such as the Shakers of New York, had already established a considerable materia medica of the "plants of the earth." As the historian Richard Hofstadter has pointed out, young America rejected formal training and credentialing as remnants of an elitist European culture.

Hydrotherapy came to America; a spa was opened in New York in 1845. Samuel Thompson, a self proclaimed healer, had already advocated steam and hot baths, since loss of heat is what caused disease. And Sylvester Graham might be regarded as an early "naturopath." due to his advocacy of the hygienic movement. Graham's "graham cracker," and John Kellogg's corn flakes were fledgling efforts to provide a perfect vegetarian food. Kellogg ran the Battle Creek Sanatorium where he advocated hydrotherapy. In mid nineteenth century America over 200 spas were operating at full steam.

One can only wonder about the steam rooms and saunas in America's health clubs today, the popularization of spas by Franklin Roosevelt, the Navajo sweat lodge, Swedish baths, the ancient Roman baths, Japanese public baths, Hippocrates advocating daily perfumed bathes, and not witness an ingrained belief by humanity in the healing power of water.

The link to American naturopathy came by way of a German immigrant, Benedict Lust (1872–1945), and his eventual association with Sebastian Kneipp (1824–1897). Father Kneipp was a Catholic priest who was prominent in the German natural healing movement, and who advocated the water cure, which he had discovered in Vatican documents. Lust contracted the then fatal tuberculosis shortly after arriving in America, and returned to Germany to await his fate. He was treated by Fr. Kneipp, regained his health, and converted to "Kneippism." He returned to America to market the water cure, first as the Kneipp Water Cure Society, then as the Naturopathic Society of America, and finally, in 1919, incorporated as the American Naturopathic Society. Lust purchased the term "naturopathy" from a New York physician, John Sheel, who had been using it to describe his personal mode of natural healing. "Naturopathy" thus becomes a proprietary term.

Lust hoped to incorporate all natural healing modalities under his umbrella organization, including the contemporary movements of osteopathy and chiropractic. He met with initial success; by the interwar period over half the states had licensed naturopathy. Long term success was another matter.

Two major forces were operating against naturopathy. One was the AMA and its refusal to recognize naturopathic colleges or their graduates. The introduction of mail order naturopathic degree programs did not help. The efforts of the AMA were largely successful, as they were against osteopathic and chiropractic at the time. The other force concerned the definition of naturopathy. It was broad enough to include a vast array of healing approaches, rendering it almost impossible to achieve consensus. After Lust's death in 1945 the movement splintered. Biomedicine reigned supreme while naturopathy lost ground.

Naturopathy is based on six principles. One, nature provides the healing power and it is the function of the naturopath to facilitate it or remove obstacles. Two, identify and treat the causes. Symptoms are not to be suppressed; they are expressions of the body's attempt to heal. Three, do no harm. Suppressing symptoms without removing underlying causes is harmful. Four, treat the whole person. Illness is viewed as an interaction of spiritual, physical, emotional, environmental, etc., factors. Five, the physician is a teacher whose duty it is to educate the patient into a healthy life style. And six, prevention is the best cure. Emphasis is on building health rather than on combating disease.

The naturopath will enlist nutrition, herbology, acupuncture, physical manipulation, all natural drugless modalities. In some instances minor surgery may be performed. But a schism exists in contemporary naturopathy. An organization known as the Coalition for Natural Health, sees the naturopath as a health counselor, not as a practitioner of medicine, and refer to themselves as traditional naturopaths. They distinguish themselves from naturopathic medicine which they allege seeks to perform surgery, dispense drugs, diagnose and treat, and, in effect, function as primary care physicians. More of this in our final chapter.

Naturopaths are currently licensed to practice in eleven states, plus Puerto Rico. In other states they function as health counselors. The American Association of Naturopathic Physicians, established in 1986, represents licensed naturopaths. It only recognizes four year graduate level residential programs. These programs culminate in the awarding of the degree of Doctor of Naturopathy (N.D.) or Doctor of Naturopathic Medicine (N.M.D.). A number of institutions offer distance learning programs in naturopathy. Some offer advanced training for health practitioners already functioning in their professions.

Doctor of Homeopathy

H.M.D. Homeopathy is a medical treatment system that is growing in popularity in the United States. After enjoying considerable success in the latter half of the nineteenth century, it fell somewhat into disrepute around the 1920's with the ascendance of pharmaceuticals, only to resurface when reports of side effects of modern drugs became known.

Homeopathy is a little difficult to handle in that it is generally associated with one of the other types of health practitioners. An M.D. may take additional training in homeopathy and incorporate it into his/her practice. Osteopaths, chiropractors, and naturopaths all may use aspects of homeopathy. So might the average consumer, in that homeopathic remedies are readily available. But these activities constitute popularized and democratized applications of homeopathy. The classical application of homeopathic techniques is quite complicated.

Samuel Hahnemann (1755–1843), a traditionally trained medical doctor, became very concerned over the move to chemical medicine that was then taking place. He further questioned the common medical practices of his day, such as bloodletting, and sought a better way.

Reportedly, while experimenting with South American cinchona bark, then used to treat malaria (it contained quinine), he noted that its use produced the symptoms of malaria in a non affected person. This observation led to the discovery of a fundamental principle of homeopathy: like cures like. The idea, then, was to find a substance that created the symptoms of a disease in a healthy person, and administer it to a person who actually had that disease. Hahnemann published the principles of homeopathy in a work entitled *Organon* in 1810.

The methodology of homeopathy involves signs, symptoms, and proving. Signs are what can be objectively assessed about a patient's condition by a physician. Symptoms are what the patient subjectively feels. And proving is trying out homeopathic remedies on healthy subjects to duplicate symptoms. Proving is the "like cures like," often referred to in homeopathic circles as "the law of similars."

Some symptoms are common to the sickness. Other symptoms are reflective of the particular individual enduring the sickness. So homeopathic remedies are customized for each patient; not all cures work the same way on every person with the same symptoms. This is termed "individualization."

Another core belief of homeopathy is that disease is a disturbance of the "vital force" or energy in a patient. Symptoms of an illness are not the illness. Homeopathic remedies are intended to stimulate the self regulating mechanisms of the body to heal itself, to restore its natural balance. The symptoms will disappear as the body is healed.

But since disease is believed to begin at the energy level, only to manifest itself as symptoms at the physical level, homeopathic remedies must not only match symptoms but energy level as well. This means that homeopathic medicine must be "potentized," that is, diluted, and "succussed," that is, shaken, to import proper energy to the substance. Successive dilutions of homeopathic remedies are known as serial dilution.

In classical or unity homeopathy, only a single remedy is to be taken at a time in order to reflect the precise condition of the patient. Hahnemannn reputedly experimented with multi dose preparations and discarded them, claiming that their use complicated the observation of the healing process. As the condition of the patient was observed as changed, a different single remedy would be formulated.

Another characteristic of homeopathic medicine is the minimum dose. The patient is to be given the very least amount of a substance that works. For homeopaths, less is better. The logic for this is that Hahnemann had observed the side effects resulting from the ingestion of large doses of powerful chemicals, and believed the minimum dose strategy was a way of avoiding side effects while maintaining effectiveness due to the "potentized" nature of homeopathic preparations.

Homeopathy was brought to the United States by the German physician, Constantine Hering (1800–1880), who is generally regarded as the "father of American homeopathy." As a medical student he was given the task of disproving homeopathy, but by successfully replicating homeopathic "proofs," as well as his personal successful treatment by homeopathy, he became a convert. Eventually, he developed what became known as Hering's Law of Cures. One, the body attempts to externalize all disease. Two, symptoms surface as part of the curative process, and appear and disappear in reverse order of their initial appearance in the body. And three, the body heals from top to bottom, and from most vital organs first to less vital organs second.

Hering moved to Philadelphia in 1833. He established the Hahnemann Medical College of Pennsylvania in 1848 and designed a "Homeopathic Domestic Kit," sort of a homeopathic first aid kit, consisting of basic homeopathic remedies for most common ailments. Homeopathy appeared in the United States at a time when the country was being ravaged by cholera, typhoid, and yellow fever. Many believed it to be an effective treatment, and it remained popular until the 1920's.

No discussion of American homeopathy can exclude James Tyler Kent (1849–1916), a conventionally trained medical doctor, who practiced in St. Louis, Missouri. Kent eventually became deeply involved in homeopathy and built extensively on the initial work of Hahnemann. His seminal work, *The Great Repetory*, is a systematic description of symptoms and cataloguing of treatments that remains in use today.

The AMA was opposed to homeopathy, as it was to all non conventional treatments at the time, but the major reason for the demise of homeopathy in the United States was the development of the pharmaceutical industry. That industry was beginning to offer numerous, easy to administer drugs that were fast acting. Homeopathy, on the other hand, was a lengthy and rather complicated process. Industrialized and urbanized America was in a hurry. Pharmaceuticals offered a quick fix.

Homeopathy remained popular in other parts of the world. With the growing movement toward alternative therapies, it has enjoyed a recent resurgence in the United States. Homeopathy is incorporated into the practices of many different types of practitioners and has become a popular home remedy. Homeopathic combinations formulated for specific conditions are now being marketed commercially. There is a National Center for Homeopathy, located in Alexandria, Virginia.

D.D.S., D.M.D. If we go by the number of practitioners, dentistry is the second largest medical field in the United States. Dental problems trace to the dawn of history. The *Papyrus Ebers* discusses tooth and gum maladies, as does also ancient Chinese texts. Anthropological remains provide ample evidence of tooth problems in early humans. The *Code of*

Hammurabi proscribes the removal of teeth as punishment for wrong–doing, a different number depending on the circumstances.

The ancient Etruscans developed dental bridges fashioned out of animal teeth, held together with gold bonds. The Hebrew *Talmud* refers to teeth made of gold, or silver, or wood. It was believed that worms caused tooth decay. In the eleventh century Albucasis wrote of dental procedures and illustrated the various dental instruments in use at that time.

During the Middle Ages, clergymen often doubled as physicians, and at the time this included dentistry. But in 1163 the Pope ruled that any procedure involving the shedding of blood was incompatible with the priestly function. So barbers began acting as priestly assistants to perform such tasks. Most tooth extractions were performed by the local barber, an early multi talented individual, who also performed bloodletting, and even on occasion cut hair. There was also a group known as "vagabonds," self taught tooth pullers, who went from village to village and performed their craft in the public square.

Guy de Chauliac, a fourteenth century French surgeon, is credited with coining the term "dentator," but a later countryman is credited with being the "father of dentistry." Pierre Fauchard (1678–1761), in his book *The Surgeon Dentist*, greatly expanded knowledge of oral pathology and procedure.

The beginnings of dentistry in America are obscured in folklore until 1734, when James Mill advertised his ability to "draw teeth." He claimed to have been trained in the art by the famous dentist, James Reading, deceased. Paul Revere made dentures and practiced the craft. Peter Hawkins, of African ancestry, was a well known tooth puller, when he was not preaching. George Washington sported a full set of dentures that were made by John Greenwood. Contrary to the popular myth that he had wooden teeth, Washington's were made of ivory, but so heavily stained due to his indulgence in port wine, that they looked like wood.

The mid nineteenth century witnessed changes in dentistry. The first American dental school was established in Baltimore in 1840. It offered a sixteen week course to train dentists. In 1851 Charles Goodyear discovered how to make hard rubber through a process called vulcanization. Rubber is moldable, and provided an excellent base upon which to mount artificial teeth. The technology was used until the World War II era. Goodyear patented the process and charged dentists a royalty to use his product. The patent was vigorously enforced until a disgruntled dentist shot a Goodyear enforcement agent. The patent was allowed to expire in 1879.

Another major breakthrough involved the introduction of anesthetics. A Connecticut dentist, Horace Wells, first used nitrous oxide for painless tooth extraction in 1844. Wells was the patient; he administered the substance to himself and had a former student extract his tooth. He named his procedure "inhalation anesthesia," and refused to patent it. Two years later a fellow dentist, William Morton, successfully used ether, and did patent it. Morton's fame spread; Wells committed suicide.

Most dental procedures require only a local anesthetic. Novacain was introduced in 1905. It was a quick acting, local anesthetic, possessed of practically no side effects. It was widely used for about forty years. Xylocaine was discovered in 1943 and has become the anesthetic of choice for most local procedures.

Just as Horace Wells had refused to patent nitrous oxide, William Roentgen refused to patent his discovery, x–ray. He made his discovery in 1895, and the scientific and medical worlds immediately embraced the new technology. A New Orleans dentist, C. Edmund Kells, is credited with being the first to use dental x–rays. This was in 1896. Kells held the film in the patient's mouth during the exposure. Like many others using early x–ray technology, Kells was unaware of the dangers of continuous exposure. He developed cancer in his hand that spread up his arm and into his shoulder. Depressed and in constant pain, he took his own life. By the 1920's x–ray had become a standard dental diagnostic procedure.

Acrylic materials made their appearance in the 1940's. UV composites appeared in the Seventies, and light cured composites appeared in the

Eighties. Lasers were being used instead of drills by the Nineties, but this has yet to become standard practice.

The American Dental Society was founded in New York in 1859. It currently has approximately 150,000 members, constituting the vast majority of all practicing dentists. It has defined its profession as evaluating, diagnosing, preventing, and treating diseases and conditions of the oral cavity and maxillofacial area. The ADA recognizes eight specialty areas: dental public health, endodontics, oral and maxillofacial surgery, oral and maxillofacial pathology, orthodontics and dentofacial orthopedics, pediatric dentistry, and periodontics and prosthodontics. Oral and maxillofacial radiology is currently under consideration as a specialty.

Standards for dental education were recommended by the Gies Report of 1926. A dentist must graduate from an ADA accredited dental school. The degree awarded after four years of standardized graduate level professional study is either the D.D.S. or the D.M.D. The degrees are identical in content; it is a matter of preference by the conferring institution. Three to four years of undergraduate work with an emphasis on science is a general requirement for admission to dental school. In some instances the fourth year of undergraduate school is combined with the first year of dental school to provide an undergraduate degree. Additional years of training are required to practice dental specialties. Educational requirements are set by the ADA. Dentists are licensed to practice in all fifty states by state licensing boards.

Doctor of Veterinary Medicine

D.V.M. Medical care of animals is an ancient concern. The *Code of Hammurabi* makes numerous references to veterinary medicine. Europeans and Asians lived with and depended on their animals, having domesticated a good number of them. Animal survival became essential for human survival. Physicians treating animals is as old as physicians treating humans.

The first school of veterinary medicine was established in France in 1761. Other institution soon dotted the European landscape. In the United States, the first veterinary school was the Veterinary College of Philadelphia, founded in 1852. The University of Pennsylvania established the first accredited veterinary college in 1883, quickly followed by Harvard. Most institutions were proprietary and established their own curriculum. If part of a university, veterinary study was usually attached to the Department of Agricultural Studies.

The United States Veterinary Medical Association was formed in 1863; its membership was small and fairly limited to the east coast. It was aware of the need to upgrade the status of the veterinarian, and largely due to its urging, the United States Department of Agriculture created the Bureau of Animal Industry in 1884. In 1898 the American Veterinary Medical Association was formed to replace the older USVMA. The idea was both to recognize the growing influence of the West in such matters. It was the president of the USVMA who recommended the change. His name was Dr. Daniel Salmon, and he was also Chief of the Bureau of Animal Industry. The emphasis of the new organization was to be educational, both for the profession, and also in matters of public health.

In 1908 the US Secretary of Agriculture announced requirements for veterinary schools, and also for veterinarians to be employed by the federal government. A joint committee made up of members of the AVMA and the Bureau of Animal Industry then rated all veterinary schools. Over the next several decades private schools closed their doors. All American veterinary colleges today are university affiliated.

The AVMA established the National Board of Veterinary Medical Examiners in 1948. Its purpose was to develop standardized licensing exams to be used by state boards. The name was changed to National Board Examination Committee in 1980. In 1994 the NBEC became a separate entity to avoid any appearance of conflict of interest (a national organization developing tests for government to use on the organizations' members). State licensing requirements are set by the states.

Many individuals think of veterinarians as individuals who meet the health needs of the family pet. While this is a function of approximately half of all veterinarians, veterinary medicine plays a major role in maintaining the health of farm animals, and a public health function in detecting and preventing the spread of animal diseases, and of animal diseases to humans (zoonoses). Worldwide concerns over issues such as mad cow's disease is but one example. Other areas of veterinary practice include zoos, the military, pharmaceutical companies, and in regulatory and inspection capacities for various agencies of the federal government.

A Doctor of Veterinary Medicine (D.V.M.) spends four years in professional training, in a combination of classroom and clinic studies, preceded by three to four years of undergraduate education. In most cases applicants to veterinary colleges possess an undergraduate degree. Internships and residencies are not required to be a licensed veterinarian, although such opportunity is available. Veterinary specialty boards began in the 1950's. To be certified in one of the twenty specialty programs in veterinary medicine a residency of two to five years is generally required.

Of interest is the fact the D.V.M. degree is particularly appealing to women. Roughly two–thirds of all current veterinary students are women, in what was once a totally male dominated profession.

Doctor of Optometry

O.D. Doctors of Optometry comprise a medical specialty that concentrates on examining, diagnosing and treating diseases and disorders of the eye. They prescribe eyeglasses, contact lenses, other low vision aids, some therapy and medicine, and in some instances, basic surgical procedures. The medical specialty of ophthalmology may perform all of these procedures in addition to major eye surgery and treatment of eye diseases and injuries.

An optometrist is different from a dispensing optician, who fits and adjusts eyeglasses according to prescriptions written by either ophthalmologists or optometrists. In some states they are allowed to fit contact lenses.

There are a number of references in ancient times to individuals with poor eyesight and no apparent remedy. During the European Dark Ages poor eyesight was not generally a pressing problem; few people knew how to read. The monks who were busy copying manuscripts, however, did have a need. Their solution was the "reading stone," a rock crystal ground into a hemisphere which then magnified. (Aristophanes had discovered the magnifying properties of glass but the discovery lay dormant.) The Chinese may have used magnifying glass for reading.

The first known definite statement concerning the existence of eyeglasses is attributed to Roger Bacon in 1268. In thirteenth century Europe only the glassblowers of Venice were capable of making transparent glass. The Venetian glassblower, Murano, is reputed to have ground glasses, and by the end of the century, eyeglasses that roughly resemble modern ones, had evolved. A reference to spectacles has been found in an Italian manuscript dated 1289.

The invention of the printing press, and its resultant increase in reading, created a much greater demand for better vision. The principle of diffraction had been formulated around 1600, leading to the invention of the microscope a few years later. The basic principles for the making of eyeglasses were then known. A charter was granted to a spectacle makers guild in 1629. Wearing spectacles was viewed as a sign of intelligence, probably due to the fact that it was generally only literate people who used them. Benjamin Franklin is credited with inventing bifocals, somewhere around 1760. Eyeglasses do not assume their modern form until around the end of the nineteenth century with the invention of the cylindrical lens.

There is a story that an English physician, Thomas Young, inserted microscope lenses in his eyes in 1801, thereby becoming the first user of contact lenses. A Swiss ophthalmologist by the name of Fick developed "contact spectacles," glass lenses placed on the eye floating in liquid. In the late 1930's the American, W. Feinbloom, discovered how to make plastic contact lenses, but World War II delayed a number of technological discoveries from reaching the marketplace. Contact lenses appeared in the Fifties.

All states license optometrists. Qualifications include a four year optometry degree from an accredited institution, preceded by at least three years of undergraduate education. The accrediting agency is the Council on Optometric Education of the American Optometric Association. Optometrists may be in private practice, work for HMO's or ophthalmologists, or work in a variety of retail outlets.

Doctor of Pharmacology

PharmD. With the growth of chemical medicine throughout the twentieth century, particularly since World War II, not only has the pharmaceutical industry become a key player in American health care, but the role of the dispensing agent of pharmaceuticals has enjoyed upgraded status as well. Pharmacists are a major component of the modern health care system.

Pharmacy evolved from chemists, alchemists, herbalists, and physicians. As medicine organized itself in Europe and the functions of prescribing and formulating separated , apothecaries were established. At first they were regulated by guilds, and later, by government. In the United States the dispensing of drugs was unregulated until after the passage of the Food and Drug Act of 1906. Everything could be purchased over the counter at the neighborhood drug store: opium, heroin, and even gasoline (druggists were the first gas stations).

In order for pharmacy to exist, first there had to be pharmaceuticals. A number of companies devoted to such a pursuit appeared during the nineteenth century. E. R. Squibb (1858) produced ether and chloroform and was a major supplier to the Union during the Civil War. Parke Davis (1867) developed the gelatin capsule. Eli Lilly dated from 1876. A German company, Merck, entered the American market in 1891. Another German company, Bayer, developed diacetylmorphine in 1898 (commonly known as heroin). In 1900 it successfully synthesized white willow bark, and called it aspirin. Various forms of pill pressing machines were designed; they were a functioning reality by the 1860's.

Pharmacology was a scientific endeavor. Discoveries had a commercial value, but discoveries required scientific research. The very nature of the industry demanded education. The first pharmacological college was founded in the United States in 1821. Absence of law and prevailing laissez faire attitudes left the public generally unconcerned with regulation. The industry itself formed a broad membership organization, the American Pharmaceutical Association, in 1852. Pharmacy became a profession when external forces changed the environment. Government regulated some imported drugs as of the late nineteenth century. The movement from over the counter to prescription drugs was an effect of the Food and Drug Acts. As the formulators and dispensers of regulated products, the status of pharmacists was elevated considerably, as well as the knowledge required to practice their craft.

After World War II, developments furthered the status of pharmacists. The pharmaceutical industry emerged as a dominant force. Paul Ehrlich had developed chemotherapy at the beginning of the twentieth century. Its central thesis was to discover synthetic chemical substances that would attack and kill specific microorganisms without harming the host body. Chemotherapy became a therapy of choice in the postwar world. Modern drugs are produced with assembly line speed. The FDA approved 160 medications and medical devices in the year 2000 alone. Twenty were classified as priority drugs. Increasingly, new drugs are more powerful, often carry associative risks, and may interact adversely with other drugs. Iatrogenic illness is a growing concern. The pharmacist has become the last line of defense in an increasingly complex chemical medicine.

Through the World War II era pharmacy students would enroll in a college of pharmacy and eventually receive a four year undergraduate degree. Internship requirements stretched the pharmacy degree to a five year program in 1960. Many institutions are now offering a variety of Masters and PhD programs in pharmacological specialties. A growing number of institutions are moving away from the Bachelor Degree in Pharmacy altogether, replacing it will a six year graduate degree, Doctor of Pharmacy (PharmD), due to the growing complexity of the profession.

Pharmacists are licensed under state law. Additionally, since they dispense narcotics, they are regulated by the federal Drug Enforcement Administration. Pharmacists generally work in retail outlets, HMO's, and hospitals. The proprietary neighborhood drugstore is disappearing from the American scene.

There are many other qualified and important health professionals, all requiring training, and usually, some sort of licensing. Physical therapists, radiologists, audiologists, registered nurses, licensed practical nurses, doctors assistants, and a host of laboratory technicians, to name a few, are all important components of the medical care delivery system. That we have not provided a descriptive account of each of these areas in no way is intended to denigrate their value and importance to health care.

Chapter Summary

- Ancient turf battles among health care professionals continue to exist.
- Allopathic medicine refers to "modern scientifically based biomedicine. The principle proponents of this type of medicine are medical doctors.
- Founded in 1847 the American Medical Association achieved major control over medical training at the opening of the twentieth century.

- Osteopathy developed due to disenchantment with the status of medical care around 1900. It is based on the principle that health depends on the structural integrity of the body.
- Osteopaths have the same training as medical doctors, but in addition, they may utilize musculoskeletal manipulative techniques, primarily along the spinal cord.
- The AMA now recognizes osteopaths and about forty percent practice conventional medicine. The majority of osteopaths function as primary care physicians and practice at least some osteopathy.
- Chiropractic developed at about the same time as osteopathy. It concerned itself exclusively with spinal manipulation, a "one cause, one cure" approach.
- The AMA was fanatic in its opposition to chiropractic, but eventually lost an historic anti trust suit at the same time that chiropractic was becoming more credible. Chiropractors are increasingly being recognized as legitimate health care practitioners.
- Naturopathy was introduced in the United States in the 1840's. Its early emphasis was on hydrotherapy, but it gradually expanded to include other natural healing approaches, and founded the American Naturopathic Society in 1919.
- Only a dozen states license naturopaths as health care practitioners. In other states they function as health consultants. Emphasis is exclusively on holistic natural healing.
- Some medical doctors undergo additional training in naturopathy.
- Homeopathy may be practiced by homeopaths, but also by any other type of health care provider, as well as individuals themselves. Based on the principles of "like cures like" and "less is better," it developed in reaction to chemical medicine.
- Homeopathy is a complicated and lengthy treatment system. The new pharmaceuticals, with their simple, fasting acting approach, easily replaced homeopathy in the United States by around 1920.

- Homeopathy is currently enjoying a comeback. This is partly due to the alternative medicine movement, and partly due to the successful scientific inquiry in to some of its long rejected principles.

- References to the practice of dentistry date from ancient times, but formal dental training in America did not occur before the mid nineteenth century.

- Dentistry has developed in to a very technical, state of the art, medical specialty.

- Veterinary medicine was prominent in the ancient world, wherein people relied heavily on their animals for survival.

- Veterinarians are generally thought of as pet doctors, but fully half are involved in agriculture and public health.

- Optometrists, in addition to prescribing eyeglasses and contact lens, treat diseases of the eye, prescribe some medicines, and perform minor surgeries. Major eye surgery is the domain of the ophthalmologist, a medical doctor specialty.

- Opticians prepare and adjust eyeglasses according to the instructions of optometrist or ophthalmologist. In some states they are licensed to fit contact lens as well.

- The pharmacist has become an increasingly important component of modern medicine and has enjoyed upgraded status.

- Pharmacists are not only dispensing agents for pharmaceuticals, but they are also federally regulated dispensing agents of narcotic substances. With increasing complexity of pharmaceuticals, the pharmacist is the last bastion against adverse drug effects.

Chapter Four

Medical Organization

From ancient to medieval times there existed no formal organization of the healing arts. Some healers doubled as religious leaders, thereby acquiring some prominence, but most quietly practiced their craft, advertising solely by word of mouth.

By the middle ages most health practitioners were self regulated, there being essentially a two tier system of healers. In villages and small towns physicians, surgeons, and apothecaries were organized along the lines of the prevailing guild system. An apprentice would be accepted by, and then serve under, a master for a prescribed number of years. He would then demonstrate his knowledge and skills before all the masters assembled, and if deemed worthy, would be granted a license to practice in his own right.

Blood letting constituted an early medical specialty, and blood letters were combined with barbers in the guild system; hence, the red and white pole. Surgeons were often incorporated into the butchering guild, the associative nature of the union being somewhat questionable. Generally, there also existed an unofficial midwifery profession, handled exclusively by women, until being usurped in some countries by the "superior male intellect" during the course of the eighteenth century. Rural areas were serviced by folk healers, both male and female, who practiced their craft devoid of any official credentialing or formal organization.

In the major cities physicians received university training, followed by the conferral of a medical degree. The value of surgery was generally denigrated at the time. Graduates would be admitted to a faculty, a college, or receive a public appointment. Local governing authorities would confer status, rights, even monopolies, not unlike the modern franchise system. Practices varied somewhat from country to country.

Early Organization or Lack Thereof

In the numerous German states, medical practitioners held medical degrees and state bureaucratic appointments. Their official duties included examining military recruits, giving expert testimony in legal proceedings, and determining sanity (although no credible criteria for doing so then existed). In France the faculties of prestigious universities were self appointed closed clubs. Individuals would receive state granted monopolies to practice in prescribed geographical areas. Intensely elitist, this medical organization was destined to become a prime target during the French Revolution.

In England the Royal College of Medicine limited its membership to Anglicans, graduates of Oxford and Cambridge only, and congratulated itself on its self created high social status, while giving scant consideration to its competency. This was certainly most unfortunate for their patients, in that the truly competent physicians were usually non–Anglican, foreign trained, or from Edinburgh, Scotland. There was a College of Surgeons, and a Society of Apothecaries, in London, but no uniform national system, and no regional licensing. Medical practice in England was generally guided by unbridled, unregulated capitalism.

Anything approaching a medical establishment in the United States simply was not to be found. American nationalism and a sense of uniqueness precluded the following of any prevailing European practice. A medical department was established at the Philadelphia Academy in 1765, and at Harvard in 1783, but democratized individualism was the name of the medical game in the young nation. American physicians, if they possessed any formal medical training at all, in all probability received it on the European continent, or in Scotland (see below). Early America was characterized by an acute shortage of trained physicians. On the sparsely populated, ever moving frontier, Americans self treated and self medicated as best they could.

Meanwhile, on the European continent, the medical center at Leiden had begun clinical training in its charity wards during the eighteenth century. One of its many skilled students was the anatomist, Alexander Munro, who founded the medical school at Edinburgh, Scotland, in 1726. This trend setting medical training center serviced 17,000 students during its first century of operation. Students could enroll for complete degree programs or specific courses. They paid for only what they chose to study. Market dynamics therefore stimulated superior instruction, while additional added value resulted from no religious qualifications, low fees, and practical training. Many American physicians who obtained their training abroad, received it at Edinburgh, partly because of the additional advantage of being able to receive instruction in the English language.

In England itself, the establishment of a private anatomy and obstetrics school in 1768, by William Hunter, was a significant event. But equally important was the advent of the teaching hospital, most likely occurring around the 1740's. The concept of clinical training, of students being in contact with patients while they were learning, was of considerable value.

The growing secularization of Europe, a development fueled in large measure by the Reformation and the Enlightenment, and the rising spirit of nationalism, resulted in the state assuming a direct role in health issues, as one way of enhancing the power of the state. The ideological precepts of

nationalism included the belief that citizens comprised a national asset—
if healthy. It followed, then, that if citizens were not healthy, they were a
national liability. It was also well documented that more casualties in the
military were due to disease than to wounds. A major movement aimed at
the safeguarding of health was the result.

Sanitation, cleanliness, maintenance of health records, and attention to
nutrition, resulted in such mundane (but at the time revolutionary) practices as bathing, washing one's clothes, feeding citrus to sailors, and gathering census data. Concomitant developments included street cleaning,
garbage collection, state sponsored hospitals, poor houses, maternity
wards, health clinics, and dispensaries. Governments were indeed assuming a very proactive role in the health of their citizenry, Medicine was
being integrated into nationalistic culture.

Nineteenth century France began with the destruction of privilege. The
aftermath of the French Revolution ushered in a brief period of laissez
faire medicine as egalitarianism held sway. But gradually, state educational
standards and licensing requirements were reinstated. The status of the
medical practitioner was strengthened, aided in no small part by the emergence of clinical hospitals. The growing monopolistic trend in the cities
gradually extended itself to the countryside. French clinical training influenced most of Western Europe.

In the German states the early bureaucratization and local licensing had
led to deregulation on the eve of German unification. The result was a
plethora of self proclaimed qualified doctors and alternative healers. The
latter were referred to as "irregulars;" the former were "regulars." Anyone
could practice medicine, the assumption being that free market forces
would drive out the most incompetent. Self appointed healers were somewhat limited by the state, but alternative medicine was, and still is, of
major significance in Germany. In 1883, however, a state medical insurance system only allowed for state payment of fees to "regular" physicians,
somewhat devaluing the role of the "irregulars."

Little change occurred in the organization of medicine in nineteenth century England. Licensing was still controlled by the colleges, often quite arbitrarily and capriciously. Physicians began to organize themselves locally, in an attempt to counteract the effects of the elitist closed system. This rather quickly led to a movement favoring national professional medical societies. The British Medical Society dates from 1855, and the Canadian Medical Association dates from 1867. The Association Generale des Medecins de France dates from 1858. Physicians worldwide sought state sponsored regulation and state sponsored monopoly. Society on a whole was not much interested in the movement.

The Medical Act of 1858 in England created a national medical supervisory board of sorts, the General Medical Council. But since the Council was dominated by the college faculties, very little change actually occurred at the time. The Act did provide for a Medical Registry of regular physicians, and contained a veiled threat of possible removal from the registry for malpractice or for consorting with irregulars. Only physicians on the Medical Registry were eligible for public appointment.

Medical Organization in Early America

Strangely enough, it was laissez faire, egalitarian America that had led the way to medical organization. The American Medical Association (see below) was established in 1847 and established standards for the MD degree in 1849. The AMA, however, faced an uphill battle for the remainder of the nineteenth century. In the American federal system the United States Congress chose not to involve itself in what was regarded as a state governmental issue. And state governments at the time were well imbued with ideas of Jacksonian democracy, which most certainly would view a medical (or any other) elite, as contrary to the basic principles of American freedom. As a consequence the practice of medicine in America was largely governed by laissez faire attitudes. These attitudes would not come under attack until the opening of the twentieth century.

In contrast with urbanized, industrialized, heavily populated Europe, wherein the governments of most nations took a proactive role in public health issues during the nineteenth century, the failure to act on the part of the United States requires some explanation.

In 1800 only a handful of urban areas could qualify for city status in the United States. The nation was overwhelmingly rural, and urban dwellers would not equal their country cousins in number until 1926. Not only was the United States rural, it was also decentralized and huge. Effective political voice and subsequent action had to await concentrated numbers, and in the case of the United States, due to its vast size, much more effectives forms of communication were needed as well.

Thomas Jefferson's writings foretold of an American nation made up of small farmers, virtuous, robust, and living in harmony with nature. The polemicists of the early nineteenth century painted a canvas replete with rugged, healthy, and happy individualists. Various essayists hammered at the difference (real or alleged) between the Old World and the New World, and most certainly the notion of a perceived decayed European culture would be rejected in democratic young America. European governmental involvement in health issues was reason enough to avoid that involvement in America.

The role of the federal government in public health issues remained near zero until the end of the century. Even then the American concept of laissez faire resulted in a government most indifferent to the plight of the working poor. This indifference would reflect government policy up to the presidency of Franklin Roosevelt. Moralistic religious beliefs and a widespread acceptance of the principles of Herbert Spencer's Social Darwinism, reinforced passive government policy. Disease and poverty were manifestations of sin, laziness, and evolution, although some religious leaders did accidentally promote a positive message when they preached the gospel of cleanliness.

Meanwhile, the cities of the east coast and the Mississippi watershed were periodically ravaged by epidemics of cholera, smallpox, typhoid, and the principle killers of the nineteenth century, tuberculosis and yellow fever. It was the latter disease, whose principle effects concentrated along the waterways and coastlines of the United States, that prompted federal action, with the creation of the National Board of Health, in 1879, the Marine Hospital Service, and its replacement, the United States Public Health and Marine Hospital Service, in 1902. State and local governments objected strenuously to these measures, but the federal government was operating under its constitutionally mandated jurisdiction over navigable and coastal waters.

The Spanish American War ended with an army of convalescents, inviting further federal action in the control of tropical diseases. The French building of a canal through Panama had been prevented, not by engineering factors, but by tropical diseases. Advances in the control of tropical diseases, in the aftermath of the Spanish American War, made it possible for the United States to eventually construct the canal.

Newly enunciated germ theory provided an impetus for public health, and as a result, the Public Health Service was established in 1912. However, the American health system, the food preparation industry, and the patent medicine industry, remained essentially unregulated at the opening of the twentieth century.

The Beginnings of Regulation

The movement of the federal government in the direction of regulation had been slow and it had been tentative. Congress passed the Drug Importation Act in 1848, the purpose of which was to inspect for possible adulteration of drugs being imported into the country. Standards, however, were non–existent. In 1862 Abraham Lincoln appointed a chemist to work for the government in the newly formed Department of

Agriculture, Bureau of Chemistry. Early government chemists quickly became aware of adulteration in the products that Americans were consuming. In 1880, another government chemist recommended that Congress enact a national food and drug law. It did not come about at that time, but henceforth, bills would be periodically introduced in the Congress. The latter third of the nineteenth century in no wise exhibited much interest in progressive or reform legislation.

In 1883, Dr. Charles Wiley was appointed chief chemist for the Bureau of Chemistry. Wiley was destined to become a tireless campaigner for national regulatory legislation. His Committee on Food Standards (1898) was influential in setting standards that would be written into the mandatory regulatory legislation that was being enacted by a number of states. In 1902, Congress passed the Biologics Control Act, ostensibly to guarantee that various serums and vaccines were safe. At the same time Congress appropriated funds to the Bureau of Chemistry to study the effects of food preservatives and food dyes on human consumption. The resultant Wiley Report was quite critical of the food preparation industry. But a recalcitrant Congress refused to act, and the Wiley Report gathered dust.

In an age wherein reform was not on the agenda of the ruling elite, by a series of unforeseen circumstances the progressive, reform minded Theodore Roosevelt found himself in the White House. Roosevelt read Upton Sinclair's *The Jungle*, a novel dealing with the sordid conditions then prevalent in the meat packing industry. The incensed Roosevelt demanded proof of Sinclair's allegations from the publisher. The proof was forth coming; also forthcoming was knowledge of Wiley's suppressed report. Roosevelt launched a public campaign encouraging people to demand that Congress pass appropriate legislation or be voted out of office. His tactics apparently worked. In June, 1906, Congress enacted in law both the Pure Food and Drug Act and the Meat Inspection Act.

During the early existence of the Food and Drug Act the Supreme Court interpreted its provisions rather narrowly, only beginning to move in a more liberal direction in the 1930's. The Bureau of Chemistry was reorganized in 1927, its regulatory functions being assigned to a new Food, Drug, and Insecticide Administration. Insecticide was dropped from the title in 1930, the name FDA henceforth becoming a permanent label.

The Federal Food, Drug, and Cosmetic Act of 1938 broadly expanded the functions of the FDA. Cosmetics were for the first time added to the list of substances subject to regulation. Drug safety testing programs were mandated, and the setting of acceptable risk standards was authorized. The setting of food standards, the establishment of inspection programs, and the power to utilize court injunctions, were also provisions of the new Act.

In 1940 the FDA was transferred from the Department of Agriculture to the Federal Security Agency, and the first Commissioner of Food and Drugs was appointed. A series of amendments during the 1940's and 1950's expanded the power and scope of the FDA. Notable at the time was the Delaney Committee, which conducted a congressional investigation of the food and cosmetics industries, and that led to the enactment of a number of additional amendments to the law. The Federal Security Agency was replaced by a cabinet level organization in 1953, the Department of Health, Education, and Welfare. In 1968 the FDA was moved to the Public Health Service.

The Federal Hazardous Substances Labeling Act, the Child Protection Act, and the Fair Packaging and Labeling Act, were all passed during the 1960's, with the FDA being charged with enforcement. The Environmental Protection Agency was created in 1970, and it was given regulatory authority over pesticides, which up to that time had been under the control of the FDA. Rather consistently over the years the FDA has had its powers expanded. But in 1976 the Proxmire Amendment precluded the FDA from regulating vitamins and minerals according to the same standards it used for regulating drugs. In other words, supplements were not to be treated as drugs.

In 1982 the FDA established regulations for tamper resistant packaging, and in the following year, Congress responded with the passage of the Federal anti–Tampering Act, criminalizing any tampering with a packaged substance. The 1988 Food and Drug Administration Act established the FDA as an agency within the Department of Health and Human Services, with its commissioner being appointed by the President. In 1992 Congress passed the Prescription Drug User Fee Act, requiring developers of drug products to pay for the cost of evaluation and approval. The monies received were to go toward hiring additional FDA staff to expedite the approval process. According to reports from the FDA the program has exceeded its expectations in this regard, while according to the FDA's critics, safety has been sacrificed in the name of speed and commercialism. The 1994 Dietary Supplement Health and Education Act granted the FDA the authority to set regulations for dietary supplements, which were classified as foods for this purpose.

Most recently the FDA has been actively involved in the anti tobacco crusade, imposing marketing and sales restrictions on the tobacco industry. The FDA has now classified tobacco as a "drug delivery device."

How is the FDA viewed? The answer depends on those who are asked. It is viewed as a defender and protector of the consumer, but it is also viewed as the bedfellow of the industries it regulates. It is viewed as an agency concerned with safety; it is criticized for its approval of dangerous drugs. It is charged with acting too fast in the approval of some drugs, and too slow in the approval of others. It is viewed as the friend of conventional medicine and the foe of alternative medicine. It is seen as both cautious and capricious. But there is one certainty: the FDA is a powerful regulatory force in American life. Most definitely, the role of the federal government in the regulation of medical care has changed vastly over the course of the past century.

Not all of the regulations pertaining to the practice of medicine were initiated by the government. The changing face of medical practice, evolving erratically, fostered scrutiny from non–governmental sources as well.

The development of scientific medicine came about slowly, resisting breakthroughs in knowledge and technique. Like most other institutions and professions it questioned change, was threatened by it, and remained essentially conservative. As it developed new insights, it did so in the absence of any unified plan. Aspects of scientific methodology began to appear, but the actual practice of medicine remained an art. Scientific medicine itself was practiced in a very spotty fashion.

The idealized "Renaissance man" was disappearing, being replaced by specialists. Specialization brought with it the positive contributions of more detailed knowledge and technique, but from a negative perspective, it ignored the whole. This led to growing institutionalization and impersonalising of medical practice. One aspect of the new scientific medicine was the appearance of research centers and laboratories. England, France, and Germany clearly were moving in this direction, the funding coming mainly from private sources.

This development was also occurring in the United States, with one very notable difference: the amount of funding available. The United States possessed philanthropists of unparalleled wealth. Influenced by the Puritan ethic, believing that one should accumulate as much as possible to fulfill their earthly calling, but equally believing that ultimately wealth had to be returned to society, individuals such as Andrew Carnegie and John Rockefeller earned billions in an unregulated and untaxed economy, then poured vast sums into medical research and other philanthropic projects.

Standardizing Medical Education

Of monumental significance were the changes that occurred in medical education during the opening decades of the twentieth century. These changes were privately initiated, multi faceted, and affected all aspects of higher education. For our purposes we will limit our discussion to those changes affecting medical education only. To understand how these changes came about, a little background is necessary.

In later life Andrew Carnegie gave away hundreds of millions of dollars; most of it went in support of educational pursuits. At the time higher education in all fields was characterized by low pay, and no pensions or benefits for professors, and no standardization of courses or programs, and no accreditation, for educational institutions. In 1905, Carnegie, having been prompted by his friend, Henry Pritchett, president of the Massachusetts Institute of Technology, created the Carnegie Foundation with an initial grant of $10 million, to fund a pension program for college professors. The following year, the Carnegie Foundation was granted a non–profit charter by Congress, and became the Carnegie Foundation for the Advancement of Education, now headed by Pritchett.

Educational institutions were required to meet very stringent Carnegie imposed standards in order to be eligible for pension funds. These included the standardization of units of instruction, the Carnegie unit, popularly referred to as the credit hour. The Carnegie efforts are widely regarded as marking the beginning of educational accreditation in America. The pension plan eventually became TIAA (Teachers Insurance and Annuity Association), the most widely used flexible plan currently in existence.

But the objectives of the Pritchett led foundation went far beyond pensions. As the name of the foundation implied, it sought to be actively involved in educational reform at the policy making level. One of its very first efforts concerned medical education.

A college preparatory school director in Lexington, Kentucky, by the name of Abraham Flexner, was given the task of investigating medical training throughout the United States, and with making recommendations for improvement to the Carnegie group. The Rockefeller family contributed toward the project. Flexner had recently written a book length criticism of American higher education, and it had catapulted him to national attention. His educational bias favored the German university model; with consistency, he also preferred the German medical model with its emphasis on research, over the English and French systems which he judged as being too clinical.

The results of Flexner's investigation were published in 1910, entitled *Medical Education in the United States and Canada: A Report to the Carnegie Foundation for the Advancement of Teaching.* It is popularly referred to as the Flexner Report. Ironically, a man who possessed no personal training in medicine would exert a tremendous influence on how medicine should be taught and practiced.

At the time American medical schools were numerous, mostly proprietary, and quite varied in terms of quality. Flexner recommended limiting medical schools to those attached to major universities only. He gave strong endorsement to the pharmaceutical and surgical approach to medicine, and recommended the inclusion of pharmacology and theoretical research in medical training. Research was to be emphasized at the expense of clinical observation. Inclusion of these new topics in formal medical training meant that certain existing topics would have to go. Herbology, natural healing methods, and nutritional studies were dropped from the curriculum.

Partly due to the fact that acceptance of the recommendations contained in the Flexner Report were made a condition for receiving Carnegie pension funds, partly because of the growing acceptance of the mechanistic view of medicine furthered by the scientific advances of the nineteenth century, and partly because both Carnegie and Rockefeller trusts were contributing heavily to pharmaceutical research, most medical schools adopted the report without reservation. The struggling American Medical Association was given the task of overseeing the implementation of the new programs, and soon became the accrediting agency for medical education, thereby achieving tremendously enhanced status.

Cooperating institutions were favored with Carnegie and Rockefeller grants. A fair number of medical schools were forced out of business, leaving only allopathic oriented institutions to provide medical education.

The immediate effect was a shortage in the supply of new physicians. Diminished supply translated in to greater demand, and this resulted in heightened status, both professionally and financially.

Flexner went on to become secretary to the Rockefeller Foundation General Education Board, and orchestrated the granting of over one half billion dollars to select medical institutions. His brother Simin Flexner, a physician, was appointed the first director of the Rockefeller Institute for Medical Research (name changed to Rockefeller University in 1965). Simon Flexner would eventually discover a serum for meningitis.

The correspondence between the brothers Flexner over the years is quite extensive, ranging from discussions on what institutions or individuals should receive grants, to who should be appointed professors at specific medical schools. Backed with huge pools of philanthropic capital, they micromanaged the direction of modern medical training. As a matter of general interest, the extensive correspondence of the Flexner brothers is housed in the library of the American Philosophical Society.

During the following decades, private capital continued to endorse and support allopathic medicine in both the United States and the United Kingdom. But it did not all come from philanthropic sources. Most well known pharmaceutical companies date from the nineteenth century, and with the move to allopathic medicine, their medical and financial importance was enhanced. The pharmaceutical industry had a vested interest in the furtherance of allopathic medicine, and began pumping its money into the new medical research centers. The efforts met with success, as many new and oftentimes beneficial pharmaceuticals were discovered. As we have seen earlier, national self interest had led to government involvement and financing of medical research during the same time period. The result was a gradually forming partnership between medicine, government, and the pharmaceutical industry, that was institutionalizing the medical system.

Certain other external forces were to further involve government in the field of medical research. Medical ethics had become a major concern by the end of World War II, as evidence of human experimentation was disclosed. This human experimentation, performed mainly by physicians of the Third Reich, led to the writing of the Nuremberg Code, which defined the ethical parameters of medical research. The later Declaration of Helsinki further defined and clarified the acceptable boundaries of medical research.

A Privatized Health Insurance System

Private medical insurance first appeared in the United States during the 1930's. Initially it was limited to the affluent, but gradually, unions embraced the concept, and medical insurance increasingly became part of a negotiated compensation package. Since employers were either paying all or a considerable part of the cost, the actual out of pocket medical costs for subscribers was minimal. Thus, the fee for service health care delivery system was easy to maintain. It should be noted also, that in the United States there were no wartime casualties, and therefore no pressing need to establish a major government role in health care for the general population. For the military the Veterans Administration and the hospitals that it operated, provided for the health needs of a specific segment of the population. The Indian Health Service and the Public Health Service also provided some limited care.

Since health insurance masked the true cost of medical care, there was a growing tendency to use it amply, perhaps sometimes unnecessarily. A healthcare culture was beginning to develop, with providers encouraging the use of their services, and with the consumer demanding more. Costs continued to accelerate, but postwar prosperity was masking the trend. For the time being the American working class was prospering, and healthcare was affordable.

But as the nation moved further from the end of the war, the traditional distribution of wealth began to slowly reestablish itself (middle class affluence eroding and being absorbed by the upper class). Some members of the middle class were beginning to be priced out of the health care market. The federal government either could not or would not intervene. The prevailing belief system equated socialized medicine with communism, and this was the era of the Cold War. Fee for service (free market pricing), financed by a myriad of private insurance plans, was the preferred course of the medical establishment. Harry Truman's brief foray into national health in 1948 met with considerable successful resistance from the AMA.

Wartime conditions had created a different course of action in the United Kingdom. The British government was forced to take over the administration of health care due to the presence of considerable civilian casualties. Government financing and government control were a reality by the end of the war, and not arguable. The move to the National Health Service in 1948, therefore, was not all that revolutionary. The new health care system nationalized all hospitals, including charitable ones. Private practitioners were allowed to continue to exist; their accessibility and personal attention offsetting their inability to provide the same degree of services available in the megalithic nationalized system. By the 1960's private practitioners had learned how to partly compensate for their limited facilities by forming group practices, and by pooling resources. Variations of socialized medicine were developed in Canada, Sweden, Germany, France, New Zealand, et cetera, but not in the United States.

Health Maintenance Organizations (HMO's) mark their beginning in 1942 with the initiation of the Kaiser Foundation Health Plan, and with the later Health Insurance Plan of New York. These plans offered complete health care programs to their members. Physicians and other health care professionals became employees of these organizations, and were rewarded for cost cutting strategies with bonuses and/or profit sharing incentives. The idea was to reduce the number of surgeries, shorten hospital stays, and perform fewer tests, ostensibly to reverse the over subscription of health services that had occurred with the advent of health insurance.

Whether HMO's provided affordable quality health care or cut corners to reduce costs and increase profits, became a matter of controversy. But what was a clearly positive development was the increasing emergence of a variety of prevention programs, "free" checkups, wellness programs, and growing health awareness on the part of many Americans.

Health care coverage in America, however, was a spotty proposition. It was becoming obvious that America's high cost health system was for the well to do. John Kennedy raised this issue but the AMA again proved itself a worthy foe. Lyndon Johnson made national health care part of his Great Society program, and in the aftermath of the Kennedy assassination, which Johnson so skillfully utilized to erect a "memorial to the fallen president," Medicare and Medicaid were launched. Under Medicare a federally financed insurance program provides basic health coverage for individuals who are eligible for social security. The extent of co–pays and limitations provide for a limited program; supplemental insurance is an absolute necessity. Medicaid provides federal funds to the states to set up a variety of health care programs for those individuals who are not covered by Medicare. In both programs the fee for service approach is maintained, but according to government imposed rates.

The continued dependence on private health insurance has made the health insurance industry and integral partner and powerful player in the delivery of health care in America. The dependence on health insurance, and the financial inability for patients personally to pay the tremendous costs of health care services, has placed the health insurance companies in the position of determining what they will pay (or not pay) and how much they will pay. A growing concern has arisen around the question of whether medical professionals or insurance actuaries are prescribing medical care. A specific health insurance plan, the preferred provider plan, does avoid some of these concerns.

As the practice of medicine became more exotic, institutionalized, and impersonal, the risks of error increased markedly. The overall effect on the status of medicine will be addressed later (Chapter Eight), but for the time being, it is to be noted that a collateral effect of error was skyrocketing malpractice insurance premiums, which would ultimately be expensed into the overall cost of the health care system. The specter of malpractice introduced a new player into the medical game. The legal profession now claims a share of the health care dollar, as attorney fees, court costs, and settlements are factored into the cost of health care.

The George Bush administration made an unsuccessful attempt at health care reform, and in the early 1990's the Clinton administration launched a multi front campaign designed to expand health care coverage. The attempt met with limited success. As the nation moves into a new administration the dominant issue has become the cost of prescription drugs. Whatever the outcome, government and medicine are inexorably intertwined.

Legal Drugs, Illegal Drugs

The national stance on drugs provides another example of the government and organized medicine working in concert. On the one hand the federal government has become deeply involved in the dispensing of medical treatments and drugs (the FDA approved 160 medications and treatment devices in 2000 alone). On the other hand the government is equally involved in preventing the dispensation of specifically targeting treatments and drugs. Opium was a widely used drug of free and legal choice throughout the nineteenth century. By the end of that century the Bayer Company had developed a synthetic replacement for it known as heroin. The principle sources to acquire these and other narcotic substances was either the physician's office or the neighborhood drug store. Little policing and even less common sense seemed to be present. The addictive nature of these narcotics was gradually recognized, but not taken too seriously. At the time addiction was simply viewed as a disease.

The Food and Drug Act of 1906 established prescription only drugs in America, and restricted over the counter sales, while the Harrison Anti–Narcotic Act of 1914 criminalized drug addiction. The byproduct of these measures was the creation of the illegal drug trade. America was on a moral crusade early in the twentieth century and national prohibition was just one aspect of that crusade. Part of the argument in favor of the passage of the Capper–Volstead Act (which enforced prohibition) concerned itself with the medical consequences of alcohol consumption. The by–products of national prohibition were bootleggers, speakeasies, and organized crime.

Following a failed concerted attempt at enforcement of prohibition during the 1920's, the nation reversed course, repealed prohibition, and focused its attention strictly on drugs. The Federal Bureau of Narcotics was established in 1930. The Bureau would provide employment opportunities for many former prohibition enforcement agents, as the moral crusade shifted focus. If anyone has viewed the 1938 government created film entitled *Reefer Madness,* the nature of government intent and government misrepresentation is readily apparent. 1937 witnessed the passage of the Marijuana Tax Act.

In 1944 a medical report claiming that there was little evidence to link poor health to marijuana use was ignored by the American Psychiatric Association, which then joined forces with the federal government on the anti drug crusade. Drug addiction was staked out as a psychiatric issue. Physicians were given the opportunity to build careers in drug treatment centers funded with government money, and legally prescribe drugs to drug users to keep from using illegal drugs.

When Richard Nixon declared a war on drugs in 1971, he had the full support of the medical establishment. Government and medicine joined ranks in creating a culture that criminalized all drug users, lumping soft and hard drugs, exempting tobacco and alcohol, imprisoning hundreds of thousands of individuals for minor offenses, and attempting to suppress a massive underground illicit drug industry while simultaneously aiding the nations supplying most of the drugs to the United States. Somehow this was for the good of humanity.

International Health Organizations

Over the course of the twentieth century, medicine organized itself on a global scale, and had little choice in so doing. Prior to the modern era, the epidemics of the world had never been truly global in their scope. Certain develops were destined to change this. Colonialism and imperialism, with their intermixing of peoples, their diseases, and their immunities, both escalated the spread of disease and contributed to the introduction of new diseases. With the development of transportation technology, increasing numbers of people move about the planet, and with increasing speed. They are all potential carriers of disease. Global commerce, the distributing of foreign agricultural and manufactured items throughout the globe, further enhance the possibility of pandemics.

The influenza epidemic that struck at the end of World War I killed twenty five million people worldwide. It was followed by a second wave, a little less deadly, in 1919–1920. The United States alone lost one half million people. The lesson was clear; in the modern world diseases could spread globally, and they could spread quickly. It was becoming evident that governments would have to pay attention to the disease issue on an international scale.

During the latter half of the nineteenth century the nations of Europe made repeated efforts to deal with epidemic cholera, seeking some international agreement on quarantine standards. It took forty one years to reach an accord that contained extremely weak provisions. In 1907 a number of European nations collaborated in creating the *Office Internationale d'Hygiene Publique,* and were eventually joined by the United States and a number of Mid Eastern and Near Eastern nations as well. Goals included the gathering of international data on communicable diseases, the development of international quarantine regulations, and the exchanging of information on a variety of public health issues.

Following World War I the League of Nations created its own Health Organization. In the western hemisphere the Pan American Sanitary Bureau dealt with health issues. Some limited cooperation existed between the two organizations. World War II resulted in a collapse of all world health institutions. Following the war, and with the creation of the United Nations, the independent World Health Organization was created.

WHO initially emphasized worldwide immunization programs and the training of supplemental health personnel. One of its programs involved a global vaccination campaign aimed at wiping out smallpox. Although this particular program was quite successful, other WHO sponsored programs to wipe out contagious diseases fell somewhat short of their mark.

The ongoing objective of a successful worldwide campaign to control infectious diseases is not particularly promising. World diseases mutate faster than counter agents can be developed. A reawakened or mutated virus can spread over the planet in a matter of days, due to the popularity and frequency of air travel, the global economy, and the manipulation of the environment. Diseases thought long eradicated have reemerged. Mass migrations of people, incessant war, refugee camps, and international workforce flow, are all contributing factors.

The AIDS virus was first identified in the United States in 1981. Its worldwide death toll is now approaching two million people. The ebola virus was discovered in 1976; it remains alive and well. Tuberculosis, once thought defeated, is making a remarkable comeback. Cholera has returned with epidemic magnitude in some parts of the world. Scientific medicine has made noteworthy advances, but it is not winning the battle.

WHO gathers health data from its 191 member nations on such issues as life expectancy, infant mortality rate, quality of health care, cost of health care, etc. It regularly develops statistical tables and charts ranking member states on a variety of health related issues. The press releases issued by WHO contain some very interesting and disturbing information. Much of its data is not widely disseminated in the American press, but it is readily available. WHO has an office in Washington, D.C., and maintains an informative website. Readers are strongly advised to avail themselves of this informative source. Some WHO reports will be referenced in Chapter Eight.

Red Cross/Red Crescent

WHO is not the only organization operating on the international scene. The Swiss banker, Jean Henri Dunant, observed a bloody battlefield in 1859, on which literally tens of thousands lay dead or dying, and on which no medical personnel were to be seen. Dunant conceived of the idea of a neutral organization to care for the wounded, and one that would also train people to handle massive casualty situations. In 1863 Dunant and four Swiss colleagues created such a relief organization. The following year the first Geneva Convention established principles for treating the wounded. Twelve nations participated in this initial effort.

Dunant's organization became known as the International Red Cross, the symbol being the Swiss flag with its colors reversed. The Red Cross became the primary training agency for nurses in those western nations that had not developed a formal training program of their own.

Eventually, 176 nations would develop national organizations, called Red Cross Societies, in all nations except Islamic nations, where they would be referred to as Red Crescent Societies. An international federation of national societies was created in 1919, in the immediate aftermath of World War I, to deal with the massive humanitarian concerns then present. The original concept of treating war wounded was expanded to include all victims of natural and human generated catastrophes as well.

In 1991 Red Cross Societies combined with all other national organizations to create the International Federation of Red Cross and Red

Crescent Societies. As the world continued to globalize, relief efforts were becoming more complex, overlapping national boundaries and political jurisdictions. In 1997 the Seville Agreement established criteria for designating a specific national organization to function as the lead agency in a particular multinational effort.

The Nursing Profession

A not to be ignored facet of medical organization concerns nursing, initially a female dominated substrata of the medical profession. The creation of hospitals had generated a need for an on site staff to handle the routine needs of the patients. Early hospitals were places to be avoided; people went there to die. As of 1800 most patients preferred to stay at home. Yet a century later, due to advances in surgery, anesthetics, antiseptics, and the increasing role of the hospital as a center of teaching, learning, and research, not to exclude the profession of medical caregivers, the nurses, hospitals had become the preferred site for medical treatment. The development of hospitals as medical care centers, however, replaced the personal doctor–patient relationship that had characterized earlier eras.

Many early nurses were provided by Catholic religious orders that specialized in care giving, such as the Daughters of Charity and the Sisters of Mercy. These organizations trained their membership for this purpose. Nursing was viewed as the material calling of a spiritual life. Such organizations performed admirably. The Protestant response was the Deaconess Institute, which trained young women to be "deaconess," or nursing sister.

One woman, who had received her training from both Catholic and Protestant organizations, was Florence Nightingale, who held the position of superintendent of nursing at Kings' College Hospital during the Crimean War. When the British press reported on the abysmal health care being provided for the wounded on the battlefield (this was the same war that affected Dunant), Florence offered her services, organized a contingent of nurses from a variety of persuasions, and headed for the Crimea. Her successes made her a national heroine, and greatly elevated the status of nursing as well.

In the United States Elizabeth Blackwell, MD, organized the nursing operations during the American Civil War, while Dorothea Dix, who had made a name for herself crusading for proper care of the insane, became superintendent of nursing for the Union Army. But it was Clara Barton, Civil War nurse, who became the American counterpart of Florence Nightingale. Barton was instrumental in bringing the Red Cross to America in 1882, and it was she who had insisted on the proviso that the organization expand its original objective and provide aid in peacetime crises as well as war.

Women have always been involved in healing. For the better part of history women's health concerns were treated by women only. The practice of mainstream medicine, however, was the domain of men. In both Europe and America in the nineteenth century, women were generally barred from certain types of education, medicine being one of them. A male dominated society simply deemed women unfit for intellectual pursuits. Some women prevailed.

The United States being a little less rigid, more egalitarian, less bound by tradition, than was Europe, broke the prevailing pattern first. Elizabeth Blackwell, previously mentioned, was the first American woman to graduate from a medical school. The year was 1849. In the following year the Women's Medical College of Pennsylvania was founded, presumably influenced by Quaker egalitarian spirit. The pioneer in England was Elizabeth Garrett, who received a certificate from the Society of Apothecaries in 1865, and later, a medical degree in France, where society was a little more liberal. Garrett would aid in establishing the London School of Medicine for Women in 1874.

In Scotland Sophia Jex–Blake battled her way into Edinburgh University in 1869, but after successfully completing her medical studies, was offered a certificate of completion rather than a medical diploma.

While the protracted legal battle progressed (which she eventually won), she acquired another medical degree in Switzerland. Subsequently, she was licensed to practice medicine in Ireland. Jex–Blake was also instrumental in founding the London School of Medicine for Women.

Minimal progress had been made by women in entering the medical profession by the opening of the twentieth century. The Flexner Report of 1910 had a negative effect for aspiring female physicians. It recommended closing many of the women's training institutions then in existence. Prestigious mainstream medical schools did not admit female students until after World War II.

There are stories of women impersonating men in order to enter the medical profession. One is of an English army surgeon, James Barry, who, on his death in 1805, was discovered to be a she instead of a he. Whether the story is true or not is begging the question. The situation it reflected was very real. One story that is verified concerns Elizabeth Garrett. She was accorded membership in the all male British Medical Society in 1874 simply because no one questioned her sex. That organization officially began to admit women in 1892.

The National Institute of Health

As a final point of information, the National Institute of Health is one of eight major agencies of the United States Health Service. It is a federally sponsored and funded agency, charged with conducting research on health issues, and with supporting research in medical schools, hospitals, private research centers, and universities. It serves as an information source for on–going research projects and clinical trials underway. The centers and institutions clustered under the NIH umbrella deal with such specific issues as aging, cancer, environment, and alternative medicine. The NIH maintains a comprehensive website, with links to a variety of government sources for heath information.

Chapter Summary

- Early medical organization and standard setting was under the control of the universities. Some governmental licensing existed, but it varied tremendously from nation to nation.

- Most early medical training institutions were privately operated and established their own curricula. Formal training in America was practically non-existent.

- Governments became involved in health issues when they began to view citizens as national assets, particularly to serve in the military.

- The nineteenth century witnessed the establishment of national medical organizations. Their goals were to promote state imposed regulation and state sponsored monopoly.

- Nineteenth century America did not follow the trend. A large, sparsely populated, egalitarian nation, coupled with decentralized government, rendered national regulation almost impossible at the time.

- Yet epidemics along the East Coast and the Mississippi waterway enabled the federal government to move into the public health arena due to its constitutionally mandated authority over coastal and navigable waters. The Public Health Service dates from 1912.

- Minimal government regulation emanated from the Bureau of Chemistry, Department of Agriculture. But its promptings led to the eventual passage of the Pure Food and Drug Act in 1906.

- The FDA has been amended and strengthened repeatedly during its century of existence.

- The relationship of the FDA and the pharmaceutical industry is held to be questionable in some quarters. Does it represent the interests of the consumer or of the industry?

- Significant changes in medicine resulted from the philanthropic activities of Andrew Carnegie and John Rockefeller.
- The Carnegie funded Flexner Report paved the way for a standardized medical curriculum based on the allopathic model.
- Legitimatization of the allopathic model was extremely lucrative to the pharmaceutical industry. It began to pour funds to further medical research in chemical medicine.
- By the early twentieth century, the triumvirate of government, AMA, and the pharmaceutical industry had institutionalized the American medical system.
- Unionization in America led to benefit packages that included health insurance. Private insurance coverage made health care widely available but also hid the true cost of medical care.
- When rising costs exceeded individual ability to afford health insurance coverage after World War II, government efforts to enter the health insurance arena were met with charges of communism.
- Extensive wartime civilian casualties forced European governments to operate their health care systems. The result was socialized medicine.
- The Health Maintenance Organization was the American response to health care delivery.
- Medicare and Medicaid provide a partial involvement of government in health care delivery. Both programs were vigorously opposed by the medical establishment.
- Private insurance companies have become major decision makers in determining health care. Malpractice issues have increasingly involved the legal profession.
- Government movement into the drug enforcement field in 1930 led to the criminalizing of some drugs while exempting others. The medical establishment was an active supporter of this activity.

- Global epidemics led to the establishment of the World Health Organization. Its initial goal was worldwide immunization. It gathers statistical data on health issues worldwide.
- Red Cross and Red Crescent Societies were created to provide neutral medical care for battlefield wounded. Services have been expanded to include all catastrophes worldwide.
- Establishment of hospitals led to a need for on-site health care givers, and the nursing profession was borne. Services were originally provided by religious organizations.
- Nursing was one medical area that was the domain of women, but some women managed to break through the gender barrier and become physicians.
- The federal government has become deeply involved in the evaluation and dissemination of health information. The major agency in this regard is the National Institute of Health.

Chapter Five

Alternative Medicine

What is popularly termed "alternative medicine" is not a new phenomenon. It appears as if both medical hierarchy and conflicting medical views have always existed. Every medical practice that has ever been considered to be mainstream had replaced a previous mainstream practice. With the advent of a new dominant practice, the displaced dominant practice would continue to exist, but in a somewhat diminished status. The displaced practice would assume one of two postures. Either it would engage in open confrontation with its successor, or it would offer an alternative. Or, as was most often the case, it would engage in a combination of both postures. This is exactly what occurred when a distinction was made between "regulars" and "irregulars" in European medical history. As long as no physician received formal medical training, there was little distinction discernible. But when formal medical training was introduced, those who did not have it became "irregular," while those who did became "regular." The former became known as folk practitioners, while the latter were university trained doctors.

Alternative medicine in the modern sense received its impetus from the advent of scientific medicine, characterized by the use of powerful pharmaceuticals, capable of serious side effects, and more intrusive medical practices than had been used in the past, notably intricate surgeries. Scientific medicine appeared during the course of the nineteenth century, heralding in a new arsenal for the war on illness. But despite the massive furtherance of medical knowledge that occurred over the century, little advantage was gained over death and disease. Not that notable successes were lacking, but the new medicine appeared to not live up to its initial euphoric expectations. So there were critics and some rejected the new medicine.

The term "alternative" is a global, all encompassing term. It can include well trained individuals and self appointed healers, authentic health practitioners and charlatans. Some alternative therapies are grounded in science, while others are not. Lumping all that is not conventional medicine into one group is a mistake, yet alternative medicine means anything that is not mainstream allopathic medicine.

The Dawning of the Medical Turf Battle

During the nineteenth century but also somewhat before, for lack of a better term, there existed the "snake oil" salesman, delivering a variety of concoctions reputed to cure everything. A susceptible and believing public seemed willing to buy in to promises of a quick and almost magical cure. The market for such remedies was particularly fertile in the United States, the one western nation that was practically fanatical in its insistence on egalitarian medical practices. Not only was the development of monopolistically based medical organization strongly resisted in nineteenth century America, but the attraction of folk medicine and natural cures seemed to possess some mysterious validity.

The osteopathy of Andrew Still was a blending of a number of pre scientific practices, into which was woven some modern scientific precepts. Various electric treatment devices, then widely sold by mail order through the Sears catalogue, were a popular therapy. The obstruction of energy flow, which the founder of chiropractic, Daniel Palmer, believed to be the source of all disease, was acceptable to the masses but not to the new medicine. The new allopathic physicians were extremely critical of these, and other, non scientific approaches.

More ethereal healing modalities were introduced through the vehicle of religious belief. Mary Baker Eddy, founder of the Christian Science faith, held that since the only true reality was spirit, and matter therefore was an illusion; all disease was an outward physical manifestation of a spiritual imbalance. At her Metaphysical College, she taught her practitioners to provide spiritual treatments for physical maladies. If the individual did not recover, it was God's will. As with all religious belief systems, there are both liberal and conservative interpretations of core beliefs. To the present day a small number of Christian Scientists refuse all medical treatment, even to the point of dying from readily treatable conditions, while the vast majority undergo spiritual treatment for the spirit, while simultaneously seeking medical treatment for the body.

Joseph Smith, founder of the Latter Day Saints, advocated only natural cures for ailments, relying on the support of Scripture for his beliefs. Early Saints were reluctant to ingest the new pharmaceuticals. Seventh Day Adventists also found the new medicine to be suspect, and initiated the naturopathic health spa in Battle Creek, Michigan. Its emphasis on clean living and proper nutrition, led to the development of the packaged cereal business. Homeopathy and hydrotherapy were popular for similar reasons.

As America moved into the early twentieth century populist medical beliefs and practices began to lose their appeal. There were a number of reasons for this. For one, the AMA was very persistent in leading the charge against unscientific medicine and in the upgrading and standardizing of medical training institutions. Buttressed by the Flexner Report, the AMA achieved considerable success in diminishing alternative medical practices. In addition, scientific medicine was aiding its own cause. The era was one of medical discovery, innovation, and advance. It appeared as if the new medicine was superior. The successes of the pharmaceutical industry seriously eroded the appeal for natural treatment. Speed, efficacy, and convenience were hard to transcend. And the federal government was moving confidently into the health care regulation arena. The presence of the Food and Drug Administration provided another powerful weapon for both AMA and pharmaceutical industry. As a consequence, interest in alternative approaches waned and would not resurface until after World War II.

Why Alternative Medicine?

The focus of this chapter is on the issue of why there even is alternative medicine, and why it is increasing in popularity. We will begin our discussion of alternative medicine by determining what it is not. Alternative medicine is not conventional (popularly termed allopathic) medicine. Conventional medicine is associated with surgery, prescription drugs, radiation, and chemotherapy as standard procedures. It rests on the principle that whatever it does is based firmly on science. It utilizes sophisticated technologies for diagnosis. It involves stringent laboratory testing. It is, by the AMA's own definition, scientifically based biomedicine.

Conventional medicine is regarded by proponents of the alternative school to be intrusive medicine. It is intrusive in the sense that its procedures, particularly surgical ones, have advanced to the point wherein the body can be treated like a machine, with replaceable parts. Many exotic modern surgeries have become routine. They are not without risk, but countless lives have been prolonged.

By its very nature modern medicine is quite expensive. Reasons for this are quite complex, and this issue will be detailed in Chapter Eight. But for the time being, suffice it to state that, within the context of our definition, scientific procedures, elaborate laboratory tests, and teams of medical personnel performing multi hour surgeries, necessarily must be expensive.

Conventional medicine is accused of treating symptoms rather than causes. There is controversy and contention over this accusation, but let us consider the following. A patient is diagnosed with a cancerous tumor. The medical decision is to surgically remove it along with adjacent affected tissue. Perhaps the surgery is followed by radiation treatments, just in case a few errant malignant cells escaped the scalpel. The process might conclude with chemotherapy. These treatments are obviously aimed at saving the patient's life; they are also aimed at treating the symptoms. What was the cause of the cancer? Certainly medical researchers are seeking answers to this question, but generally, conventional medicine treats the symptoms of disease, not the cause of disease.

In all fairness here, many allopathic physicians will advocate appropriate life style changes for their patients—diet, exercise, weight reduction, and so forth, but more often than not after the patient has recovered, not as a standard preventive approach. However, most patients do not seek out an allopathic physician because they want to map out a program of healthy living; rather, they seek one because they are ill, and more often than not, they want a quick fix. Most patients want to have their symptoms treated. Underlying causes are far less important than feeling better. Allopathic physicians treat symptoms of illness because, one, this is what they have been trained to do, and two, this is exactly the type of treatment most of their patients prefer.

This is not a criticism of conventional medicine. It is doing what it is designed to do, and in most instances, within its self–imposed parameters, it does an excellent job. Allopathic medicine has saved many lives. Its treatments have prolonged many others. It is a much desired and important medical modality—appropriately used.

Recently conventional medicine announced that the routine prescribing of antibiotics for influenza patients should be discontinued. The rationale for such prescribing had been to provide a precaution against possible secondary infection resulting from the flu. But it had long been known by individuals both inside and outside the medical profession, that the more antibiotics are administered, the less effective they become.

Conventional medicine is based on germ theory. Invading pathogens cause disease. But recall the controversy over germ theory and terrain theory mentioned in Chapter One. Conventional medicine is germ theory oriented. Understand, however, that germ theory versus terrain theory is not an absolute either–or scenario, with the adherents of the two positions lined up 100 percent on one side or the other. Alternative medicine emphasizes terrain theory, that is, build up the immune system so the pathogen cannot do its dirty work. Truly informed alternative practitioners recognize when allopathic treatment is the correct one. If a patient is suffering from a raging infection, debating over germ versus terrain is rather absurd.

The AMA has imposed rigorous standards for the training and educating of medical practitioners. Those standards are formed on a "scientific basis." What is not scientific is to be spurned. Clearly, science is a major driving force in the modern world. But there could be a problem with, as the old saying goes, "putting all one's eggs in the same basket." Let us retreat for a moment to the time when the scientific method was being formed.

How Scientific Is Science?

For millennia humans had wallowed in fear and superstition, and the source of both was ignorance. Not knowing what caused various natural phenomena, they attributed causes to demons, angry gods, and spells. So when certain basic discoveries were made concerning the laws of the physical world, it was indeed liberating. The figure of Isaac Newton loomed large over the pages of the seventeenth century, and casts its shadow on the twenty first century. Newton and his contemporaries discovered that the material world was governed by physical laws. Discovery of these laws eventually would lead to understanding, and through understanding control would be achieved. Discovery meant delving deeply into the nature of things. It meant taking things apart; seeing how they worked; putting them back together; seeing if they still worked. It meant formulating a theory, testing it, by quantifying, measuring, and observing.

A systematic way of going about research was certainly a most positive step toward knowledge and understanding. But science is a product of its own level of understanding. When the steam engine was placed on a set of wheels on parallel rails to create the first rudimentary railroad engine, scientific pundits claimed that the device would disintegrate at thirty–five miles an hour. Nothing could go faster than that! The 1940's era computer pioneers were predicting national needs for two, or three, or maybe even four computers. When IBM did a market feasibility study for its proposed Tape Processing Machine in 1951, it estimated eventual sales of twenty–five units. Physicists working on the atomic bomb were concerned that once a chain reaction was begun it might not be stopped. They went ahead with the tests anyway. If a man could fly he would have wings. Tell that to the aircraft industry. The speed of light is an absolute value in the universe. Then researchers fired a proton 200 times the speed of light by altering the field through which it was fired. Change the conditions, and change reality. And most recently, some astrophysicists claim that the speed of light has changed over time, challenging the absolute value of Einstein's famous equation. So much dogmatism can hardly be termed science.

Science is supposed to seek knowledge, objectively and rationally. Science is to be conducted with an open mind, yet time and again, science is dominated by unbridled dogmatism. Seek not the truth; rather, seek to protect one's own turf. Scientific objectivity has definitely yielded greater knowledge. But emphasis on itself is, in itself, not objective. Knowledge is acquired both objectively and subjectively. The two modalities comprise a balanced set of opposites. But scientific objectivity has denigrated subjective knowledge. The subjective nature of humanity is suppressed in order to worship at the altar of objectivity, which, due to its growing dogmatic nature, is hardly what it claims to be.

The very application of science, in its reductionism, is leading to some very disturbing discoveries. Science presupposes a mechanistic universe, subject to rigid law. Yet delving deep into the nature of things has uncovered a reality in which none of Newton's laws seem to apply. Quantum physics has discovered a reality that is plastic. The experiments of the renowned world physicist, Dr. Leonard Mandel, indicate such mind boggling results as: protons have no definite characteristics or any reality before being observed; an unmeasured quantum system resides in potentiality until it is observed; light is both particle and wave.

Is there any validity beyond scientific objectivity? Can truth be known subjectively? Is "vitalism" (life force) a concept to be scorned? Neurophysiologist Norman Allan researches in the area of "patterned water," that is, water that remembers what substance was put in it after the substance is removed. The suggestion is that the serial dilution process of homeopathy, which seems to defy science, can be proven by science. Reality is dotted with anomaly; Einstein's theory of relativity is an anomaly. In its application science "proves" contradictory observation.

A commonality seems to exist among creative people. If one reads the biographies of scientists, inventors, composers, mathematicians, engineers, etc., overwhelmingly the solution to the project they were working on came to them in a dream. Is this a scientific way to obtain knowledge? Science is quantified; therefore, it should be predictable. In biomedicine, when a certain stage of an illness is reached, a predictable event is supposed to occur. Usually it does, but sometimes, it does not. Explain scientifically a spontaneous remission of disease. Numerous studies have been done on the power of mind, of emotion, and of placebo effect. They consistently indicate that there is a level of causation outside of science.

Science: The Projection and the Reality

Science and technology have never completely delivered on what they promised. Early scientific discoveries resulted in euphoria; humankind would discover all the laws that governed not only nature, but human institutions as well. The ultimate result would be indefinite progress—a veritable utopia on earth.

Adam Smith "discovered" the laws of economics that resulted in capitalism. A host of thinkers "discovered" the laws of government, that found expression in the political experiment known as American democracy. The introduction of the factory system was to provide efficiency, raise the standard of living, provide extensive consumer goods, end backbreaking labor, and yield considerable leisure time. The introduction and marketing of numerous home appliances were justified on similar grounds.

Substantial improvement in the quality of life would be the result of science. So mass culture jumped on the bandwagon of science. Validity was to be found only in that which was scientific. . Therefore, the study of government became the study of political science, social studies became social sciences, and the art of medicine became scientific biomedicine.

There is no arguing that industrialized, democratized nations possess a higher standard of living than do less developed societies. But did we get the utopia that was promised? With hundreds of billions of dollars spent on programs to eradicate poverty, disease, and ignorance, have these conditions been eliminated? Science was overly optimistic.

As has been discovered, science is only one of the players on a highly crowded and interactive field. Special interests, turf battles, politics, economics, environmental concerns, religious beliefs, etc., all affect its application. But if none of these complicating factors were present, there would still be a major problem for science.

Scientific discovery does not come about without a price. The personal automobile is indeed a wondrous machine. It provides ease of travel, convenience, mobility, and it provides congestion, pollution, and expense. Air conditioning is quite pleasant, but then science discovered the effects of chlorofluorocarbons and ozone depletion. The verdict is still out on the effect on humans by radio waves, television signals, microwave ovens, and cell phones. High voltage electrical transmission lines lose five percent of their power in transmission, and there are claims of subsequent health problems for cattle and for humans. Every one of these technologies provide positive features, yet the long–term effect of their use is not known.

New technologies have a habit of affecting people and society in a number of unanticipated ways. The sleeping pill, thalidomide, the insecticide, DDT, and the diet drug, Fen–Phen are the products of modern science, and science initially regarded these products as safe to use. Science was very, very wrong. Atomic power generating plants are great, even though they were originally proposed as a cheap source of electrical power that never materialized. And then came Three Mile Island, and later, Chernobyl. All these scientifically derived products and procedures cost money. The promised leisure, then, is generally sacrificed to earn the money to buy the things that were supposed to create more leisure. Society has experienced unbelievable social and cultural change as a byproduct of science, the long–term effects of which are yet to be determined.

The delivery of American medical care now absorbs fifteen percent of the Gross National Product, more than twice that of any other nation in the world. A little over one hundred years ago the cost was close to zero percent. There obviously has had to be a massive redistribution of financial resources. A byproduct of technology has been the creation of the service industry. All those wonderful technological gadgets require maintenance and servicing, and people have to be paid. The overall cost of living in technological societies is escalating. Whereas humanity once wallowed in misery, it can now be cynically claimed that science and technology has enabled humanity to be comfortable while it wallows in its misery.

The Psychology of Change

Another issue in the growth in popularity for alternative medicine is change, and the psychology of change. Natural changes, such as the process of aging, or changes in the weather, are generally regarded as normal parts of living. But change in the patterns or routines of life as we have established them for ourselves, is oftentimes not so readily accepted, and indeed, may be viewed with apprehension or even fear. The reason, simply put, is fear of the unknown. The present, even if it is miserable, is known; the future is not. The distinction for many is crucial, and some creative and predictable behaviors are the result.

Change may follow a normal progression to acceptance. At first it is categorically and violently opposed. With time opposition mellows to toleration. Eventually, opposition is dropped and the change is embraced. Previous opposition is then denied and erased from history, and credit might even be claimed for originating the idea in the first place. Modern medicine is very good at "discovering" things that alternative medicine has known all along. For a long time the holistic approach was denied by conventional medicine; patients were dismissed with such admonitions as "its all in your head," something that alternative healers readily accepted and used as part of their diagnosis and treatment. But when it was eventually "proven" that there is a mind–body connection in health and disease, conventional medicine took credit for it. Equally is this true with nutritional supplementation.

Change, historically, breeds its antithesis. The more rapidly and broadly it occurs, the more people romanticize about the "good old days." Nostalgia is a great defense against change. The consequence can be a Luddite (anti technology) type resistance to change. Modern medicine has changed so much in recent decades that part of the move to alternative medicine can be attributed to it. There is far less anxiety associated with the familiar, with the natural. Imposing diagnostic equipment operated by nameless technicians can be very threatening to the patient. The alternative approach, on the other hand, generally involves a non invasive one–on–one personal relationship.

Impersonality

The impersonality of modern conventional medicine is an issue. It operates at a factory pace. More time is spent with the house painter discussing complementary color schemes than is spent with the physician who is prescribing powerful side effect ridden pharmaceuticals. This is a very real factor; the servicing of allopathic medicine leaves something to be desired. Did you ever swear to never return to a restaurant because you received lousy service, even though the cuisine was quite excellent?

One characteristic of science is its reliance on quantification. It measures, counts, tabulates, and develops statistical data. It also sets standards for what it terms "acceptable risk." By its very methodology it does not provide absolute assurances of success. Science is fallible. There is a five percent chance one might develop side effect X. There is a forty percent chance the procedure may cause condition Y. There is a ten percent chance one might die in surgery. People become percentages, numbers. Can you get more impersonal than that?

American society has changed massively since the 1960's. Use whatever term you like: Now Generation, Baby Boomers, Yuppies, Self Gratification Society, individuals today are much better informed, more assertive, less elitist, and less traditional than the generations that preceded them. All of these changes affect how they view medical care and how they treat medical practitioners.

The information revolution is certainly a factor. Availability of information, even for the somewhat less technically sophisticated, has never been so extensive. The deadening effect of pabulum television is well documented, but television also presents many very informative and educational programs for those interested, including programs on health and science. One can actually watch surgeries being performed on television. Some of the investigative reporting type programs provide worthwhile information in a form readily understandable by practically anyone willing to view them. Knowledge has been popularized and democratized.

News magazines and specialty magazines provide in depth reports that are not compressed by the time demands placed on newspaper accounts. There has been, without exaggeration, an explosion of magazines devoted to health issues. Overwhelmingly, the health issues discussed are alternative health issues. On the other hand, few people read *The Journal of the American Medical Association,* or the *New England Journal of Medicine,* nor are their articles written for any reader audience other than a professional one.

Web sites devoted to health issues abound, and there is considerable variety. Government sponsored web sites present updated information on conventional and some alternative medicine. Alternative medicine sites do likewise within their areas of specialization. The web can be used to research a disease, seek out treatment options and locations, and find a physician. Health questions can be posted on a number of web sites, or discussed in numerous chat rooms. Tremendous amounts of information are readily available. There is a caution however. As all experienced web surfers are well aware, not everything on the web is correct information. It is essential to research carefully, double check, verify from other sources, and not blindly accept any information, from the web or from any other source as well.

Related to the impersonality issue is what futurists refer to as the human need to compensate for high technology. There was a time when most daily activities were interwoven with social function. For instance, a bank deposit involved an interaction with a live person, one that you might get to know personally over a period of time. There was a time when an actual living person put gasoline in your car, washed the windshield, checked the oil, and perhaps performed minor automotive repairs. He worked in or owned the neighborhood "filling station," and you actually knew his name. These simple interactions added value to life.

In the two examples just given, an ATM transaction has replaced human interaction. Across the span of human activity this is increasingly becoming the norm. Wherever it is possible to substitute automation for a human being it is being done. In the process, personal relationships are obliterated. Equally is this true regarding modern medicine practice. Speed, efficiency, and technology, all in the name of science or economics, has replaced the personal relationships that once existed. At one time the physician was a personal friend, knew the entire family, and advised and consoled. No more.

The compensatory activity for impersonal high technology involves a retreat from technology to more basic human needs: human interaction. Ironically, call in talk shows, chat rooms, support groups, various New Age activities, counseling groups, etc., are all manifestations of the need to replace what technology has taken away. So too, I believe, is the growing trend toward alternative medicine.

For alternative medicine is not high tech; it emphasizes the "natural," and it is holistic. It emphasizes dealing with the patient as a person. The very nature of the alternative approach calls for the attending physician to get to "know his/her patient. There have been studies that indicated that elderly people sometimes visit their physician not because they are ill but because they are lonely. They do not require a pill; they need a symbolic hug. People need to interact with other people; sensory deprivation is debilitating. If they cannot interact within the scope of their daily activity, then they will seek out other alternatives.

In natural healing part of the healing process is psychological, emotional, relationship based. Feelings do affect recovery. Negative individuals become ill more often and recover more slowly than positive people. Why are conventionally trained physicians "amazed" at a spontaneous healing or remission? Alternative practitioners are not amazed; they expect such occurrences as the norm. And why? Theirs is a different paradigm.

Alternative Cultures, Alternative Medicines

"Celebration of cultural diversity" is a frequently quoted expression. The United States is and always was a multi racial, multi ethnic, multi cultural nation. Cultural diversity cannot be sorted into neatly defined categories. Diversity knows no boundaries; one cannot accept only part of a culture and still champion cultural diversity. One cannot pick and choose which parts of a culture one chooses to celebrate. It is a matter of all or nothing, all the beliefs, including its medical beliefs. One effect of the national championing of diversity has been a growing toleration and interest in alternative therapies from different cultures.

It should therefore not be surprising that there is a resurgence of Chinese medicine, Ayurvedic medicine, Native American medicine, and Islamic medicine. Interpretation of "political correctness" dictates that society should show respect for all the beliefs of all the people, regardless of their foundation in fact. In the process, individuals become acquainted with medical treatments that possess an appeal, either because they are new, strange, or mysterious, or because they seem to work. The reason for the attraction really does not matter. The opportunity to come into contact with new or different medical practices is a part of the modern cultural milieu.

As global economy increasingly becomes reality, as people travel more widely and more frequently, it is not only the dances, songs, and wines of the world that are being discovered, it is the medicines of the world as well. It is not only our food that comes from around the globe, it is our nutritional supplements as well. Noni juice from the South Pacific, herbs from the Amazon rain forest, herbs from China, oils from the Mid East, and various glacial drinking waters, are but some examples of this new and globally diverse phenomena.

Social changes have also had their effect on how we view our medicine. People once deferred to and respected authority figures. This never was a rigid behavior because the pull of anti elitism has always been strong in America, and class consciousness has never developed to the level that it has in many other nations. But "The Movement," the social revolution of the 1960's, changed the manner in which we treat each other. Individual rights were discovered, rights were demanded, and rights were flaunted. Decorum gave way to the new value of personal assertiveness. The early feminist movement embraced "assertiveness training." It became socially acceptable to announce pride in oneself, in one's heritage, race, culture, gender, ethnicity, life style.

The permissiveness that resulted from Sixties behavior led to an emphasis on self–gratification, the "me" generation. The Beatles proclaimed that "Love is the answer," but another side of the era indicated otherwise. People became more aggressive, more self centered, and more assertive. A competitive and aggressive nature is admired in American culture. The rise of American capitalism was buttressed by Social Darwinism. The cult of spectator sports is based on winning. The drug addicted entertainer and the dysfunctional millionaire athlete are tolerated, even excused, as long as they are star performers, if they can win.

Part of the "I got my rights" mentality is evidenced by the growing number of people viewing their medical care differently than they once did. Doctor–patient relationship smatters of a superior–inferior relationship. The patient today views medical care from the viewpoint of consumer. The consumer is in charge, and the health provider is the consumer's employee. Many modern health care consumers know what they want (television drug ads are a prime source of created need), demand what they want, and if they do not get what they want, they seek another physician. The docile, passive patient is slowly disappearing. The growing commercialism of modern medicine is counterbalanced by the growing consumerism of the modern patient.

The changes of the Sixties brought about a rejection of the traditional parent–child archetype, of which doctor–patient is an aspect. When the movie *Mash,* first appeared, it was vigorously opposed by the AMA, for the movie portrayed doctors as being very human; the façade was under assault. The celebrated Shepard murder trial was viewed as particularly egregious by the American public because Shepard was a physician, and physicians simply did not do such things. A trust had been violated. A number of pedestals were lowered in the Sixties: politicians, religious leaders, health practitioners, and most other traditional authority figures. A cynicism emerged from the revelation that these people behaved like everyone else. The status of privilege was to be no more.

In some measure this changed perception was the inevitable culmination of the American popularized interpretation of democracy. Equality before the law, which is what the United States Constitution guarantees, somehow became equated with equality of skill, talent, and knowledge. The goal was one of finding the lowest common denominator of mass America, and making it the norm, popularly referred to as the cult of mediocrity. Knocking the elites from their pedestals was somewhat vindicating, and a vicarious pleasure was thereby derived. Pulling you down is far easier than raising me up.

Egalitarian Beliefs

But a more positive dimension involves a legitimate freedom, that being the right to choose. What separates a democracy from other types of political systems is the degree of personal freedom allowed to exist: the freedom to choose a career, friends, location, life style, even one's preferred medical treatment. This is significant. The freedom to choose is a fundamental right. For a society to deny that right is to make a mockery of democracy, yet there is a concerted attempt by some to do just that.

It is interesting to note that those who would impose their system of behavior on others seem to consistently fail to realize that by so doing, they are often actually reinforcing that behavior. Tell people they cannot do something, and some, out of defiance will do it, even though they initially had no intention of doing so. The consumption of alcohol did not diminish with the enactment of national prohibition, but it did make criminals out of people for doing what they had always done. Tell people they cannot partake of their supplements of choice, and most assuredly, many will find a way. What is legal is what a legislative body, a court, or a government agency states is legal. What is legal is not necessarily what is moral, or what is right.

Contrary to big government mentality, there are many people who do not seek and do not want the government in their daily lives. They really do prefer to take care of themselves. We see this preference expressed in many avenues of life, not only in the area of health care choices. Increasingly, people are forming self help groups, support groups, health food cooperatives, and community outreach groups. They are growing their own organic food, preserving the environment, becoming less energy dependent, and relying on each other rather than on the government. The home schooling initiative is an aspect of this, as are neighborhood associations, block watch programs, and community policing.

Personal Empowerment

The aforementioned moves stress independence, they are empowering, and they partially compensate for the growing impersonality of modern culture. One obvious way of avoiding or at least minimizing the effects of modern culture is to implement appropriate life style changes. In the field of health care the most effective life style change is the one that emphasizes prevention. Nutrition, dietary supplements, and exercise programs are somewhat reminiscent of the health spa movement a little more than a century ago.

Interest in the holistic approach to mind–body is at an all time high. Meditation techniques, relaxation exercises, spiritual classes, theosophy classes, and metaphysical schools, provide ongoing opportunities for people from all walks of life. People are searching for answers in a mechanistic impersonal world that some refer to as an insane asylum. Critics frequently refer to those interested in such things as "New Agers." But the same caution applies to the so–called New Age Movement as does to alternative medicine: there is no one–size–fits–all definition. Many very sincere and responsible people are seeking order and control in their personal lives.

Thirty years ago the consumer had to seek out a 'health food' store. But today, due to increased demand (and the market follows demand), there are health food stores in every shopping center and strip mall. Every other shopping center sports a health club. Memberships in health clubs, enrollments in yoga and t'ai chi classes, the use of dietary supplements, and the purchase of home exercise equipment, are all evidences of a health conscious trend and self–empowerment.

Consumption of hard liquor has diminished nationally, tobacco use has dropped (at least for older Americans), people are increasingly concerned about maintaining their health by avoiding unhealthy practices or situations, and by building the immune system of body. The intent is to perhaps avoid the impersonal HMO, the hurried specialist, or the toxic drugs. These behaviors conjoin extremely well with the philosophical framework of most alternative medicine. Devotees of the natural movement are very concerned about the side effects of pharmaceuticals, the risks of surgery, and the limitations of scientific biomedicine. Theirs is not a blind faith; they seek other, or more complementary, approaches.

Some of the reluctance to partake of modern medicine involves a growing wariness about the limitations of modern biomedicine. In some respects modern medicine has overstated both the alleged infallibility of science and the successes of its own treatments. While quick to challenge the "proof" of alternative medicine, conventional medicine has rarely "proved" the efficacy of many of its own treatments. Instead, it assumes itself to be superior, because it has determined that its scientific paradigm is superior. What is the "cure rate" for conventional medicine? For alternative and complementary medicine?

The Apple and Orange Comparison

The issue is complicated by the fact that it is impossible to obtain and compare data since the *modus operandi* of the two approaches is so different. Conventional medicine concentrates on disease, while alternative medicine concentrates on health. If an individual pursues a healthy life style, and then evidences good health, is the good health the result of the life style or genetic structure, or luck? Can an alternative approach be credited with the preservation of health? Also, are most cures the result of medical intervention, or is the body curing itself? Is belief in the treatment, regardless of its type, more important than the treatment itself. Some studies have indicated that as many as thirty percent of patients receiving placebos are "cured."

There is a growing confidence gap. Medical mistakes appear to be increasing, and if they are not, then at the very least, the publicizing of them is increasing. It makes people wary. And some medical positions do appear a bit absurd. When an article in a leading medical journal states that the incidence of breast cancer can be reduced by removing breasts before they become cancerous, and no one is laughing at this preposterous suggestion, we have a credibility gap. Why not just kill everyone who is healthy and thereby prevent them from dying from a disease!

And finally, there is evidence that many alternative therapies are grounded in science, and that they do work. Science is uncovering scientific validity for popular folk culture treatments, and it is discovering the intricate interrelationships that exist at the quantum level of physicality. It is becoming increasingly difficult to categorically deny anything (see Chapter Seven).

The federal government appears, at first glance, to have become far less rigid in its stance on alternative medicine. Through the National Institute of Health, one of the eight major agencies of the United States Public Health Service, it established the Office of Alternative Medicine in 1993. At the time the OAM was placed under the Director of the NIH, and it possessed a rather limited budget. In 1998 Congress replaced the OAM with the National Center for Complementary and Alternative Medicine, as a full center within the National Institute of Health. Its budget was increased substantially.

The charge given to the new national Center, is to rigorously apply scientific research to determine what complementary and alternative practices and treatments work, which do not, and why they do or do not work. The Center evaluates herbal products, nutritional supplements, and vitamins, as well as treatments such as acupuncture and chiropractic. Furthermore, the Center trains the researchers of complementary and alternative medicine in the proper research methodology of biomedicine. The Center also possesses a major charge in the area of communication.

NCCAM maintains a Clearinghouse, established in 1996, which provides information to the general public on complementary and alternative issues. Information is available by telephone, fax, through various internet databases, news releases, and on request, through its many publications. All information is available free of charge. Instructions on how to access all aspects of NCCAM information can be gotten from its extensive website.

The existence of NCCAM appears to be a definite positive one. To some extent this is true, but there is a fundamental flaw in the program. Science espouses objectivity, but the accepted standard of excellence for the NCCAM is biomedicine. The only acceptable methodology for evaluating complementary and alternative medicine is the methodology of biomedicine. The inherent assumption, then, is that biomedicine is not be questioned; it is the Absolute. Complementary and alternative medicine is only valid if it fits the biomedical model.

Complementary and alternative medicine is being evaluated according to the standards of a mechanistic scientific model that reflects modern biomedicine. Evaluating non–mechanistic modalities with the tools and standards of the mechanistic mindset, simply does not make any sense. These standards are based on an interpretation of reality formulated over three hundred years ago. They imply that our understanding of physicality as determined then has remained static, and this is hardly the case. If you build an instrument that measures light within a certain frequency range, it will not recognize light outside of that range. It will only measure that which it was designed to measure. If you have a belief system that is programmed within prescribed limits, it will not operate outside of those limits. Commonly referred to as in–the–box thinking, it precludes creativity and innovation, out–of–the–box thinking. Most individuals hold their beliefs so rigidly that even to casually question them is not an option.

When Galileo revealed his observations on the nature of the solar system, the established authority of his day, the Church, which was devoid of any knowledge of science, applied the standards of the Church in evaluating the correctness of his discovery. Galileo's monumental discoveries were repudiated, and condemned as heresy. The Keepers of Truth throughout history have always imposed their rigid beliefs on new ideas.

There is some worthwhile information available through NCCAM. Just understand that it has been filtered, and only what can fit in a predetermined scientific "box" is acceptable.

Chapter Summary

- What can be termed "alternative" predates modern scientific medicine. The dispute over what is the "best" treatment has always existed.

- American egalitarianism fostered a climate that produced a wide variety of populist medical practices up to the early twentieth century.
- By using pharmaceuticals, surgeries, radiation, and chemotherapy, conventional medicine has been labeled "intrusive." Since it does not utilize these treatment modalities, alternative medicine is regarded as being non intrusive.
- The emphasis of conventional medicine is on treating symptoms. The emphasis of alternative medicine is on treating causes.
- Science provides the validation for conventional medicine. Yet science possesses its own shortcomings, and is currently valid only within a narrow band of reality.
- All scientific advances come at a price. Sometimes that price is unanticipated disaster.
- Change is rigorously resisted by those who have much invested in the status quo. Change is rarely embraced by society in general due to a fear of the unknown
- The institutionalization and specialization of conventional medicine renders it very impersonal.
- There is a need to compensate for high tech impersonality with human interaction. This is something that alternative medicine claims to provide.
- Interest in alternative medicine is partly the result of the diversity of American culture, and partly the result of the globalization of commerce and knowledge.
- Since the Sixties Americans have been much less willing to accept the pronouncements of the "expert" unchallenged.
- Since the Sixties a segment of the population has been much less willing to accept responsibility for their own actions.
- At the same time there exists a national movement of individuals seeking to take control of their own health.

- There is a crisis of confidence in the medical establishment due to the growing awareness of the severity and frequency of medical errors.
- Alternative medicine is becoming increasingly validated by science, yet remains humanistic and personal.
- Alternative medicine is slowly moving into the mainstream of medical practice, but government seeks to control it according to the standards of conventional medicine.

Chapter Six

Phytomedicine

Phytomedicine is the term used to describe medicines or other healing substances that are derived from plants. It comprises the oldest form of medicine, and eventually evolved into herbology. An herb is a flowering plant, the stem of which does not become woody. The plant may be a food plant, a medicinal plant, or it may be poisonous. We are concerned here only with those plants that possess medicinal properties.

Different parts of the plant possess different healing properties. Some plants were named after that particular part of the human body for which they seemed to have the most beneficial effect, for example, liverwort or eyebright. Crude plant extracts were most likely the first medicines, generally consisting of leaves, roots, stems, and occasionally, the fruit. The plant material may have been ingested raw, cooked, or boiled, and it may have been applied topically, in the form of compresses. Plants were often processed into tinctures or teas, and used singularly or in combination. Crude plant materials can be prepared homeopathically to enhance their effect, but this most certainly was unknown to ancient peoples.

Scores of books have been written that contain detailed information on herbs, herbology, and herbal medicine, so there is little to be gained from a reiteration of this information. In this chapter we will concentrate on three uses of plant materials. The first to be considered is the relatively new field of phytonutrition. The other two are concerned with more subtle and esoteric derivations of plant material: flower essences and essential oils.

Phytonutrients

The late twentieth century witnessed the appearance of phytonutrients. The word phyto refers to plants, while phytonutrient refers to all of the phytochemicals, minerals, vitamins, enzymes, etc., that naturally occur within the plants.

When we ingest plant material we normally ingest only part of the plant. If we ingest phytonutrients we ingest some of the entire plant material. The theory is that we thereby receive the benefit of all of the components that make up the plant, rather than just a few isolated components. The theory further holds that when all of the plant components are ingested together, they act synergistically, that is, the sum of the parts exceeds the whole. Much greater nutritional value is obtained from each component in the plant when taken in combination, than would be obtained if taken singularly. This holds true for all plants, whether they be fruit, vegetable, or herb.

Early pioneers in the health field movement were just that—pioneers. They were taking the first steps into uncharted territory. Their emphasis at the time was on what was just beginning to be know at the time. Vitamins had recently been discovered, the role of some minerals and some amino acids was known, but an understanding of the interaction of various nutritive substances in the body was in its infancy. Knowledge of enzyme activity existed, but was certainly not widespread.

Dietary supplementation with these substances was regarded as an important adjunct of good health. But with the passage of time, due to continuing scientific research, it was discovered that there were many other nutritive components, and these were needed to prevent imbalance in the body. Supplementation with specific substances could lead to deficiency of other substances due to the delicate balancing system of the body. Early nutrition researchers were realizing that the application of scientific reductionism to nutritional components, if that meant taking specific isolated substances, could have unfortunate consequences. So the move toward whole plant foods was the result.

Initially, efforts were directed toward singular plants: barley, alfalfa, wheat grass, chlorella, and spirulina, which were highly charged, naturally occurring nutritional substances. Substances were purchased in powder form, mixed with juice or water, and ingested singularly. In the process the entire array of plant material was being ingested as a whole food. What is interesting about these "green drinks," is the fact that, in addition to their extraordinary combination of natural nutrients, they are also natural antioxidants and deodorizers as well.

Over time a number of reputable companies would begin to formulate whole food products that were a combination of a variety of naturally occurring foods. In addition to whole plant materials from a variety of plants, high fiber concentrates and prebiotics, diary–free probiotic cultures, and such additional natural foods as bee pollen, royal jelly, soy lecithin, and a variety of herbs and extracts, would be added.

Continuing laboratory research has discovered direct links to certain phytonutrients and the prevention of disease, suggesting a growing importance of these substances for health. The advent of super phytonutrients is all the more important when one considers the dead foods that are increasingly being offered to the American public, foods that are the products of depleted soils, chemical agriculture, and over processing and adulteration. Genetically altered foods do not address the problem; they compound it. Genetically altered foods will increase quantity, but at the expense of tampering with naturally occurring quality. Science and commercialism insists on knowing more than nature. We are what we eat.

Phytomedicine

Some herbs, such as dong quai, red clover, black cohosh, etc., are referred to as phytoestrogens, or, natural estrogens derived from plant sources. It is believed that phytoestrogen herbs yield estrogen–like effects, binding to estrogen receptors in the body, but without raising estrogen levels, which is widely regarded as a dangerous event. It is further believed that phytoestrogens mimic the effect of low level estrogen in the body without creating the side effects normally associated with the taking of synthetic hormones.

The *Journal of the American Medical Association (JAMA),* in a year 2000 article, stated that hormone replacement therapy resulted in a 53% increase in the chances of contracting breast cancer. It would seem that one should consider her options on this issue. A very informative book on the subject is Raquel Martin's *The Estrogen Alternative.*

There is a category of herbs known as adaptogens, a term first used by a Russian medical researcher in 1947. Adaptogens are natural plant materials that aid the body in maintaining homeostasis, or balance. This suggests that they would be particularly effective for stress related conditions, but they have also been proven to be immune enhancing. Adaptogens aid the body in coping with, or in learning to tolerate, certain stressful stimuli, and this eventually increases the body's resistance to that stimuli. Various types of ginseng, ginkgo biloba, golden root, and St. John's Wort, are examples of adaptogens.

The quality, and therefore, the subsequent effects of the use of all natural products may vary. Where a plant was grown, what the soil and climate conditions were at the time, when it was harvested, and how it was processed, are all determining factors. It is important that the consumer self educate on the company's from whom they purchase their natural products.

Phytoremediation

Phytoremediation is the process by which living plants can be used to correct environmental pollution. While we are on the subject of plants, and since environmental hazards are a major factor in health, some mention should be made of this new technology.

Plants can remove a variety of toxic substances from soil and water. Some plants absorb heavy metals from the soil; they are known as hyperaccumulators. Other plants degrade various organic compounds by utilizing their own enzymes and bacteria. Research is underway to discover which plants have the greatest capacity for absorbing radioactive contamination.

Phytoremediation is inexpensive, at least when compared to other types of environmental cleanup. It leaves the cleanup area relatively untouched: no bulldozing, stripping of soils, etc. On the negative side, it takes time to clean up an area in this manner, usually two or three growing seasons. Further, the plants that are used to suck up all the bad stuff in the soil are themselves contaminated. They contain very high concentrations of the contaminated material. They can readily and inexpensively be disposed of, but at issue is whether animals and insects will nipple on the contaminated material in the meantime, thereby corrupted the entire food chain.

Nevertheless, phytoremediation offers an interesting and promising solution to one of the modern world's greatest health concerns. At issue is simply determining which plants work for a particular contaminant. Plant use may well be the future of ecological engineering

Flower Essences

Flower essences are the result of the lifelong research of Edward Bach (1886–1936), a medical doctor and naturalist. Similar to other far thinking individuals, Bach was concerned about the shortcomings of medicine as it was being practiced in the early twentieth century. Over a period of time, through persistent observation, Bach reached the conclusion that the personality of the patient was actually more important than the disease in the treatment of the patient. The same treatment that worked on some patients did not work on others with identical symptoms. Therefore, it was the patient and not the disease, and more importantly, the attitude of the patient, that was to receive primary consideration. For Bach, life and health was expressed by harmony and balance; disease was the product of disharmony and imbalance. He believed that nature, in its infinite wisdom, had provided the cures for all ailments.

In May, 1930, Dr. Bach reached the conclusion that the morning dew that had settled overnight on flower petals must contain some of the essence of the plant. Collecting the dew from the petals of flowering plants, and subjecting it to a variety of experiments, Bach reached the conclusion that dew exposed to sunlight was far more effective than dew that was not. Somehow the sunlight helped energize the essence of the flower into the dew.

Collecting workable quantities of dew from the petals of flowers was, however, a rather grueling and impossible task. So Bach collected the petals themselves, placed them in bowls of water, exposed the bowls to sunlight, and let nature do the rest. The result was uncontaminated plant essence. Bach believed that the flower contained the absolute maximum plant energy; after all, it contained the concentrated energy needed to reproduce. The sun exposed water was believed to contain an ethereal imprint of plant energy. In effect, an energy pattern had been created.

Bach stored his flower tinctures in small bottles, using sparing quantities of brandy as a preservative. Through a lifetime of experimentation, he determined which flower essences worked best with specific moods. He believed that disease could only be cured by treating its cause, and the cause was ultimately the mood of the patient, not the symptoms being expressed. Treat the mood; the cure would follow. He believed that his flower essences contained positive energy that counteracted the negative energy that produced disease.

During his abbreviated life Bach discovered thirty–eight "soul" qualities and thirty–eight corresponding flower remedies. Somehow disease was seen as the result of a disconnection between the personality and the soul in some specific quality. The energy essence of the flower remedy reestablished the connection. In addition to his thirty–eight flower essences, all of which were single flower tinctures, Bach developed one blend, Rescue Remedy, widely used to alleviate the effects of traumatic situations. Bach's Flower Remedies are known worldwide.

His remedies consist of natural products indigenous to his native British Isles. Other researchers from other parts of the world have built upon his pioneer research. Numerous single essences and blends are the result of the globalization of flower essence research. There are now product lines of essences representing plants indigenous to all parts of the planet. The use of flower essences consistently over a period of time are believed to restore subtle energy bodies, and many cures have been claimed as a result of their use.

Essential Oils

Another approach to obtaining the maximum energy from a plant is that of extracting the lifeblood of the plant. By pressing or by distilling, the essential oils of a plant can be extracted, yielding some potent therapeutic substances and subtle energy medicine effects. Interest in, and the use of essential oils, has reached explosive proportions in recent decades.

The rediscovery of these plant essences in the twentieth century has led to the creation of the general term "aromatherapy" to describe these essences, many of which possess very distinctive and powerful scents. In the popular mind aromatherapy is associated with scented candles, perfumed bathes, and various forms of massage, but these associations are far from complete.

The study of the essential oil of plants, or aromatherapy, is not the same as the study of herbology. References to plants and herbs in ancient texts do not, therefore, necessarily refer to the oils of these plants and herbs, although the possibility certainly exists. The practice of herbology may involve use of the entire plant. Essential oils are strictly the essence of the plant. Herbs, particularly in their dried form, can last indefinitely. Essential oils, if not properly stored, are perishable.

Herbs were the first medicines of the masses. Often they were coarse, bitter, and generally unpleasant to ingest. But they were relatively inexpensive and quite plentiful. Oils, on the other hand, were processed, and consequently, much more expensive, less plentiful, but certainly preferred over herbs by those who could afford them.

Essential oils are very versatile substances. They may be applied topically, inhaled, diffused, and many may be ingested. They have been used since ancient times as medicines, cleansing agents, scenting agents, food flavoring, and in massage. They played a major role in early religious rituals, although much of early scenting was due to the burning of the resins of plants. The true scope of the therapeutic effects of essential oils is only beginning to be known. A unique characteristic of essential oils is that their constituents can be determined scientifically, making it possible to establish rational links in determining their efficacy. It is for this reason that some leaders in the essential oil movement prefer to use the term "essential oil science" instead of "aromatherapy" as more concisely defining their unique nature.

The Spice Trade

One of the widely known commercial endeavors of the ancient world was the spice trade. Recent research indicates that ancient peoples were quite mobile, and the overland trade routes across Asia are well documented. Long before the Christian era the Chinese had established contact with the East Indies, trading heavily in the Spice Islands. Ceylon was the first major trading center in the East; later, another would be established in southern Arabia.

Caravans were regularly moving a variety of spices, resins, and gums, including cinnamon, frankincense, ginger, tumeric, myrrh, cassia, and cardamom, to the ancient Mid East approximately four thousand years ago. The Arabs would eventually develop sea routes and become the first middlemen. Alexandria was destined to become the major port of entry in the Mediterranean world for a variety of aromatics, but the Arabs continued to dominate the spice trade until the time of the Crusades.

The Crusades, partly religious, partly economic, and partly political, marked the first tentative step in Europe's eventual worldwide expansion. Europe was introduced to the wonders of the East and the Italian city–states became the funnels through which eastern goods entered the European world. The Italian city–states were simply the last link in a chain of middlemen stretching to Asia. It was largely due to a desire to cut out all the middlemen that Europe set out to reach the spice rich countries of the East directly.

By the sixteenth century the ships of Portugal, Spain, England and Holland, were plying the East Indies. In the seventeenth century France would join in the quest. The ships of these nations reached the East by sailing around Africa. Columbus sought a more direct route, sailing to the west. The accidental "discovery" of America by Europe was the product of the European quest for the spices of the East.

It Is a Scented World

Scents were undoubtedly discovered at some unrecorded time through the simple process of smelling. Living in a natural environment, early humans possessed highly developed sensory capabilities, as these were essential for survival. Some scents were found to be pleasant, others not nearly so. We are only beginning to understand the intricacies of scents, how at the subconscious level they affect our emotions, or even our attraction or lack thereof, for other individuals. Sensations were probably associated with certain scents through a process of trial and error. Modern research indicates that certain scents trigger specific biochemical responses. A smell once experienced is never forgotten; nor are the circumstances under which it was experienced ever forgotten.

At some point an aromatic plant was accidentally crushed or pressed, and it released its liquid fragrance. It was discovered that the liquid could be rubbed on the skin, and that the fragrance would continue for some time. It was probably further discovered that the liquid plant essence could be saved for future use by storing it in a closed container.

The burning of aromatic plants in all probability occurred by accident. An aromatic plant was thrown on a fire as added fuel, but gave off a strong fragrance mixed in the smoke. These smoke laden fragrances appeared to have certain mystical or magical effects on people. Subsequently, the smoking of aromatic plants, or the burning of incense, would become quite widespread in the ancient world. And since certain fragrances created a mind or emotion altering effect, they were associated with the supernatural, and became integral parts of religious rituals. "Smoke houses" are still used in the health practices of some cultures, and smoke ceremonies are part of many traditional religious ceremonies. The use of incense in some contemporary religious rituals owes its origin to these ancient practices.

Many animal species mark their territory with scent, rely on their sense of smell for safety, track their evening meal by scent, and are attracted to breed by scent. Canines are attracted to eat not by taste, but by smell. Some of these traits seem to be present in the human gene pool. The human digestive process is stimulated by positive food odors. Recent research suggests that a great deal of human sexuality is associated with the interaction of subtle scents. There is absolutely no question that smell has a direct and profound effect on the human organism.

The first oils used were those that came from plants containing high concentrations of fatty oils, such as olive oil, linseed oil, and sesame seed oil. None of these oils possesses a strong scent. They were probably used as carrier oils, that is, strongly scented substances were blended into them.

Essential Oils in the Ancient World

Ancient Egyptians were very much concerned with cosmetics. Skin crèmes, ointments, and coloring agents were widely used by around 2000 B.C. Vases discovered inside the tomb of Tutankhamen contained residues of fats combined with frankincense. Over three thousand years ago the content of these vases would have been in a more liquid form. Egyptian physicians mixed oils, herbs, and other less savory substances as cures for various ailments. Egyptian priests offered incense and oils to their gods.

Overwhelmingly, the oils used in the ancient world were fatty oils, to which were added such aromatics as myrrh, frankincense, and cedarwood. Whether the Egyptians possessed knowledge of the distillation process is arguable. Recent archeological finds along the Pakistan–Indian border have uncovered devices that resemble stills. They date from around 3000 B.C. Another device, clearly a still, was discovered in Afghanistan, and it dates from around 2000 B.C. Whether these devices were used to distill essential oils is not known; it is a possibility. In any event, even if the process of distilling essential oils existed in the ancient world, it would have been used very sparingly. The most widely used forms of aromatics were gums and fatty oils. The *Papyrus Ebers* makes mention of oils, but the only ones mentioned by name were the fatty oils. A large number of aromatic plants are mentioned, but it is not specified as to their form.

In the *Book of Exodus* Moses is instructed to mix a number of specified herbs in olive oil to produce an "oil of holy anointment," to be used strictly as an oil of consecration. Likewise, Moses was instructed to make a perfume (incense) from certain prescribed herbs and it, too, was to be used only for religious purposes. Aromatics were used in the purification rituals of Hebrew women, as a deodorant, and apparently, even as an aphrodisiac.

Aromatic waters were apparently widely used by the Greeks, but especially by the Romans. Herodotus, a famous Roman historian, chronicled the crushing of aromatic plants, soaking the material in water, and then using the water on the body. It appears as if the perfuming of the body, by both men and women of the upper classes, was widely practiced. Scent distinguished classes; the upper classes smelled of perfume, while the lower classes smelled of sweat (presumably members of the upper class did not sweat). Some writings suggest that there were medicinal benefits that were to be derived from the use of perfumes. Recipes for medicinal perfumes have been discovered carved into the walls of Greek temples.

It was the Romans, with their preoccupation with public health issues and public baths, who embraced aromatherapy. Perfumery was a very big business in the Roman Empire. The Romans used oils, ointments, and scented powders, and the tonnage of aromatic substances imported annually from the Mid East was substantial. The Roman world was a scented world.

It is highly likely that the Germanic tribes who displaced the Roman Empire and were destined to populate Europe, brought with them a folk medicine. They had come out of the East and in their travels, certainly had acquired knowledge of natural substances. What is beyond speculation is the fact that their contact with Roman legions introduced them to aromatics. Roman soldiers carried seed pouches of aromatic plants with them on their extensive military campaigns. The plant knowledge of the East filtered through to the Germanic invaders largely through Roman civilization.

Short term it probably mattered little. The collapse of the Roman Empire in the West brought about a period of retrogression for Europe

(Gaul). The achievements of two principle underpinnings of western civilization, Greek and Roman, were buried. The early Christian church, the only surviving legacy of the late Roman Empire, declared surviving Greek and Roman works to be of pagan origin, and ordered them destroyed. Europe lost its origins and considerable accumulated knowledge in the process.

Learning languished in the West, but continued to flourish in the Mid East, where the Eastern Roman Empire (the Byzantine Empire) was destined to survive for another one thousand years. Arab culture would preserve and study surviving Greek and Roman texts, in effect becoming the guardians of western culture. The only evidence of learning in the West was provided by the Carolingian Renaissance (early ninth century), and by the clandestine copying and preserving of surviving manuscripts, work going on across Europe behind monastery walls.

Europe had retrogressed. The hygiene, public baths, and public health regulations of Roman days disintegrated, to be replaced with disease, filth, and plague. Superstition and witchcraft dominated the belief system, while demons and sorcerers were said to roam the land. Dynastic wars prevailed, only adding to the misery that was all too commonplace. It appeared as if Europe had to almost totally emasculate itself before the building of a new civilization could begin.

The Islamic World

The Islamic world was a world of fragrance. By the ninth century it appeared as if the Arabs had mastered the distillation process, although it may have occurred much earlier. There is evidence to the effect that the Japanese had developed a similar technology in either the seventh or eighth centuries. Avicenna, who is generally given credit for inventing distillation, more likely simply improved on an already existing technology. Definitely, by the ninth century, essential oils were in widespread use in the Arab world. Oils were used as medicines, in religious rituals, and in baths. Indian, Chinese, Japanese, and Arabian texts dating from the end of the first millennium all reflect extensive use of oils and aromatics.

Arabian perfumes and essences were well known in the Mediterranean world, which suggests that they were being produced in sizeable quantities. Distilled essences and fragrant waters were brought to Europe during the time of the Crusades. Whether due to knowledge acquired from the Arabs or independent effort, various aromatic "healing waters" were developed by various cloistered religious communities around this time. St. Hildegard has been credited with inventing lavender water (twelfth century).

The Arabs had made notable progress in alchemy, thereby providing the basis for chemistry. One notable achievement involved discovering how to distill alcohol (an Arab word), which, when combined with aromatics, created the perfume industry. It was no accident that the European perfume industry began on the Italian peninsula, in the Venetian city–state. Scent became the rage of the Italian upper classes, who carried scented balls and wore scented clothes. Catherine d'Medici carried the custom to France when she married the French king, and France quickly embraced perfumery. From France scents would pass to Elizabethan England

Renaissance Europe and Beyond

Aromatics were widely used as a protective shield during the many plagues that scourged Europe. The burning of piles of aromatic woods was a common practice when the plague was present. Infected buildings were fumigated with a concoction of aromatic substances. Incense was burning everywhere; scented candles were ever present in the sick room. Perfumed substances adorned the body.

Europeans were doing what they could to cope with a difficult situation. They lacked a scientific basis for the use of aromatics, but they did seem to help. Essential oils especially, but aromatic herbs as well, possess antiseptic properties. Of note was the fact that the perfumers themselves, those who were constantly immersed in aromatic substances, were scarcely touched by the effects of the plague. And the unsavory characters of the era, those who robbed the sick and dying, protected themselves from contagion by dowsing themselves with aromatic substances.

By the thirteenth century the works of Dioscorides (see Chapter One) were circulating through Europe. By the fourteenth century English texts began to occasionally mention infused oils (the English initially used infusion whereas the French and Italians used distillation to extract their oils), and by the fifteenth century, knowledge of oils in England was widespread.

In the later middles ages Europeans rarely bathed and seldom washed their clothes. Previous mention has been made of the aromatic world of the Arabs. The European world was also an aromatic world, but considerably less appealing. Early indigenous American descriptive accounts of Europeans, as chronicled by Spanish missionaries, repeatedly commented on the foul odor of Europeans. To some degree the widespread popularity of perfumery in Europe was due to its ability to at least partially mask the effects of poor hygiene.

Those who could not afford perfume (it was expensive) derived what benefits they could from aromatic plants by "strewing," that is, spreading cut aromatic plants on streets and paths so that as they were stepped on and crushed, they would release their aromatic (or deodorant) properties. It was common to plant aromatic plants around homes, as a rustic medieval lawn, again, to be tread upon, releasing the essences trapped within.

One of the unforeseen consequences of the Age of the Crusades, with its reacquaintance with its Greco–Roman past, was a movement known as the Renaissance, or rebirth. Whereas the preceding period had been dominated by religious themes in art, architecture, and literature, the Renaissance celebrated humanity for its own sake. Disassociating themselves from the confining thought of the medieval period, Europeans now considered themselves free to investigate the material world and what it had to offer.

Contact with the Mid East brought about another development. The Arabian world believed in comfort and pleasure. Silk clothing, spices, and exotic foods were commonplace, and clearly the antithesis of European coarse clothing, bland food, and monotonous diet. Contact also stimulated interest and practice in alchemy in the European world.

Alchemy to Chemistry

Alchemists were viewed as fringe scientists They possessed knowledge of distillation, using it regularly in their craft, but they also used spells, incantations, and astrology, in seeking the elusive "philosophers stone," an alleged secret process that would convert base metals into precious metals. But alchemists did make many significant discoveries, and these discoveries provided the foundation for the modern science of chemistry.

By the very nature of what they did, and the techniques that they employed, alchemists would be considerably involved with essential oils. A particularly fertile environment was found in the German states. By 1597 Jerome Braunschweig, a physician, compiled a list of twenty–five essential oils, along with these medicinal uses. By around 1700 essential oils were being used extensively for medicinal purposes.

The seventeenth century had begun with a rash of inventions that made possible the precise observation of the physical world. Galileo, Descartes, Kepler, Hooke, Boyle, Leibnitz, and of course, Isaac Newton, the reputed father of the scientific method, were of that century. Robert Boyle, in the 1660's, laid the foundation for modern chemistry, and Newton, in the 1680's, formulated the laws of a mechanistic universe.

At the time both herbs and essential oils, in fact, all natural medicine, was being prepared by apothecaries (forerunners of modern day pharmacists), who possessed knowledge of distillation. With the advent of the chemical approach to medicine advocated by Hohenheim, which received considerable status enhancement from Robert Boyle, physicians had a choice to make: prescribe the traditional herbs and oils, or adopt the new chemical medicine.

So although the end of the seventeenth century witnessed the common medical use of essential oils, with prescribed doses and uses clearly delineated, and with the likes of the English physician, Nicholas Culpepper's *The English Physician*, expounding the merits of essential oils, a counter movement was underway. Physicians were beginning to prefer the standardization, the alleged reliability, and the quick action of chemical drugs over natural products. Herbals were prescribed less and less, eventually passing from use. Initially, essential oils continued to be used by both herbal and chemical oriented physicians, but with gradually diminishing incidence.

During the course of the eighteenth century essential oils continued to be discovered and researched. By the middle of the century over one hundred oils were in use. Up to that time the oil industry was unified; regardless of the use to which they were put, they came from the same processing source. But by the 1860's cosmetic fragrances split away from essential oils and synthetic chemical fragrances were introduced. The cosmetics industry would overshadow essential oils for the succeeding half century.

In 1910 the German chemist, Otto Wallach, received the Nobel Prize in chemistry for his work in identifying and analyzing the chemical compounds in essential oils, notably terpenes. Led by France, research in the properties of essential oils would continue, and eventually, France would restore the former medical connection of the oils. And for this development credit must be given to Rene–Maurice Gattefosse (see below).

Oils in the Twentieth Century

One of the side effects of early industrialization and urbanization was the growing prevalence of contagious diseases, particularly tuberculosis. At one time the disease affected a significant portion of urban populations, particularly in areas where there was substandard and crowded living conditions. It has already been pointed out above that aromatics had seemed to ward off the effects of plague, and the same can be said for tuberculosis. It seemed that the workers who tended, harvested, and processed the aromatic plants used in the French perfume industry, did not contract the disease. The fact that many of these workers spent their day in an open, somewhat healthy environment was certainly a factor. But the observation of the phenomenon led to the first laboratory testing of the properties of essential oils. The date was 1887.

Since 1887 there have been literally hundreds of scientific studies pertaining to the efficacy of essential oils. It is ironic that, at the very time when there was an explosion of accurate information pertaining to essential oils, mainstream medicine elected to ignore the data. Oils were used medically at a far greater incidence when their value could only be empirically observed and speculated upon. With the advent of hard data that indicated the relationship of the chemical components of essential oils with curative effects, one would expect a resurrection of interest in and use of the oils. But such was hardly the immediate result.

A number of studies during the late 1800's demonstrated the antibacterial effects of cinnamon, cedarwood, sandalwood (biblical oils), juniper, thyme, and lavender. The disinfectant and antiseptic properties of clove, chamomile, and lemon were discovered around the World War I era. In general, however, the information drew little attention. It is to be recalled that this is the same time when chemical medicine is becoming dominant, and the general public and the medical profession both were marching to the beat of the new drum.

The pivotal figure in the rediscovery of essential oils was Rene–Maurice Gattefosse. The story on how he became interested in essential oils appears in every single book on aromatherapy. And since it clearly was a watershed event, it will be retold again.

The Gattefosse family owned a perfume business, not a unique enterprise for a French family. Gattefosse was trained as a chemist, and worked in the family business as an investigator of the properties of essential oils from the perspective of cosmetics. He noted, during the course of his research, that the oils he was working with as part of his family's business, possessed better antiseptic properties than the new chemical antiseptics that were appearing in the marketplace. But at the time, the information did not seem to have a profound effect on him.

Gattefosse experienced an unfortunate mishap in his laboratory, and one hand was rather badly burned. The often repeated story is that he plunged his burned hand in a vat of pure lavender oil, thinking it was a vat of water. He is said to have experienced almost immediate relief from pain, and the burn healed quickly with no scarring. It is now known that lavender oil exerts significant positive effects as a treatment for burns. The incident launched Gattefosse on a lifelong investigation of essential oils. He is credited with coining the word "aromatherapy," or, a therapy based on treatment with aromas.

The research into the properties of essential oils by Gattefosse remained relatively unknown for several decades. An individual who was acquainted with the therapeutic properties of essential oils was Dr. Jean Valnet, a World War II era French army surgeon, who, in the absence of traditional medical supplies, made use of the essential oils in his treatment, in that they were available in his native France. Trained in medicine, Valnet noted the positive effects of the oils. After the war, Valnet, and a biochemist, Marguerite Maury, popularized the work of Gattefosse.

Valnet's book, *Aromatherapie,* was translated into English in 1982 under the title of *The Practice of Aromatherapy.* Along with the Englishman, Robert Tisserand's *The Art of Aromatherapy,* an American edition of which appeared in 1985, aromatherapy was brought to the attention of the American public. Over the course of the past two decades a host of authors from England, France, and the United States, and other countries as well, have written extensively on the subject of aromatherapy and the chemical components and therapeutic effects of essential oils.

Properties if Essential Oils

In the next chapter we will discuss the various facets of energy medicine. The premier energy medicine of the ancient world was essential oil. By definition essential oils are volatile and aromatic liquids extracted from plants through the process of distillation. Some of the oils are extremely volatile, meaning that their molecules vibrate very rapidly (rose oil has the highest volatility), making them excellent natural sources of energy medicine.

Essential oils contain the highest known levels of oxygenated properties of any natural substance currently known, as well as naturally occurring negative ions and ozone. Essential oils are anti bacterial, anti fungal, immuno stimulating, nutrient transport enhancing, and possess an electrical direct current frequency that is harmonious to the body. Analysis by gas chromatography has revealed the presence of hundreds of different chemical compounds in some oils. The possible combinations of compounds for positive synergistic effect are astronomical.

Whereas viruses mutate to counteract the effects of antibiotic drugs, no known virus is capable of mutating against the effects of essential oils. Ongoing research by medical doctors in Europe (where essential oils are mainstream treatment options), and a growing number of open minded health professionals in the United States, are documenting the properties of essential oils, utilizing widely accepted research techniques.

The properties and characteristics of essential oils, and the various therapeutic uses to which they can be applied, are well covered in scores of books that have been written on the subject in recent years. It will serve no useful purpose to rehash that ground. But all oils also possess a frequency. In light of rapid developments in the new field of energy, or frequency, or vibrational medicine, this aspect of essential oils deserves attention. The discussion will also serve as a bridge to the next chapter

Oils and Frequency

The study of frequency was not possible before the advent of the scientific age. This is an energy universe, and all matter consists of nothing more than concentrated, integrated energy patterns. All material objects consist of vibrating molecules, and therefore, emit a specific and discernible frequency.

A number of individuals during the course of the twentieth century have investigated and experimented with frequency related healing modalities. In most instances such activity has been shrouded in mystery, intrigue, litigation, and conspiracy theory. A case in point concerns the life and work of Royal Raymond Rife, scientist extraordinaire.

Rife believed that every biochemical compound possesses its own distinct frequency. Everything that physically exists has its own distinct electromagnetic signature. Therefore, Rife reasoned that if the precise frequency of a disease could be determined, and then altered, the disease would be destroyed because it would cease to be itself. Exposing a diseased organism to its own frequency (which Rife in some unknown manner modified) killed the disease with no apparent side effects. (For a discussion on Rife and other pioneers in the field of energy medicine, read the section on Radionics, Chapter Seven.)

Rife's approach is based on using instruments to create frequencies. Research in the field of essential oils suggests that similar results could be achieved naturally, that is, simply by using the oils. The essential oils of plants possess a much higher frequency than the plant itself, and this is why oils are listed as volatile substances. Many oils have a much higher frequency than the human body, with rose oil being the clear leader (at 320 hertz). The theory is that by ingesting, inhaling, or topically applying oils the frequency of the body will be raised.

Research indicates that negative emotions lower body frequency, and further, that the use of high frequency oils raises body frequency, and has a positive effect on emotional and spiritual centers. Perhaps this accounts for the ancient development of incense for use in religious rites.

Diffusing specific oils has different effects. Some oils are particularly effective as disinfectants or antibiotics, while others may aid in achieving mental clarity. Individuals highly skilled in essential oil science can blend various oils to enhance particular effects.

Recently (mid 2001) an Australian pharmaceutical company "discovered" the long known and well documented antiviral, antibacterial, and antiseptic properties of oils as a weapon to be used against hospital acquired infection (which has been done in western Europe for some time). They have produced a revolutionary new "drug," available only to physicians and hospitals, that appears to be a blend of specific oils. How did blended oils become drugs?

Chapter Summary

- Phytonutrients are all the nutritive components that naturally occur within the entirety of a plant.
- Early phytonutrients were mainly single plant "green drinks," but have evolved into health cocktails of natural food substances.
- Some plants appear to possess medicine like effects without the side effects of chemical medicine.
- Plants may also provide a solution to environmental issues. The use of plants absorbing toxic substances is known as phytoremediation.
- Flower essences are believed to be concentrated plant energy as found in its petals, captured and energized in water by exposure to sunlight.

- Specific flower essences are believed to exert positive healing effects on specific conditions.
- Use of flower essences is regarded as a subtle natural energy approach.
- The original flower essences of Edward Bach were indigenous to the British Isles. Flower essences are currently derived from worldwide sources.
- Aromatherapy was widely known in the ancient world. It was used primarily in religious ceremonies and in the practice of medicine.
- Immense demand for aromatics led to the Spice Trade, and later became the main factor in Europe's geographical expansion that resulted in the discovery of the New World.
- Since fragrances were seen as affecting emotional and spiritual centers, they became an integral part of religious ceremony—through the burning of incense and anointing rituals.
- Oils are frequently mentioned in ancient manuscripts; they are found in the tombs of prominent individuals who had packed items of value for the next world, and in a number of scriptural references.
- The Greeks perfumed themselves, the Romans took aromatic bathes, but with the collapse of the Roman Empire, all such practices temporarily ceased.
- Oils were widely used in the Arab world. Knowledge of oils and alchemy were combined with discoveries in chemistry. This information was passed on to Europe.
- Aromatics were widely used to protect against the effects of the plagues that ravaged Europe.
- By around 1600 knowledge of essential oils was widespread in Europe. Oils were an integral part of medical treatment.

- The move to chemical medicine, and the use of oils mainly as cosmetic agents, led to the demise of the therapeutic use of oils until the twentieth century.
- Ironically, scientific investigation validating the properties of essential oils occurred at the same time that oils were being repudiated by conventional medicine.
- Rene-Maurice Gattefosse is created with reviving interest in essential oils and with coining the term "aromatherapy."
- Aromatherapy did not receive major attention in America until the 1980"s.
- Essential oils exhibit a number of characteristics that make them excellent sources for natural healing.
- The volatility or frequency of oils (this is what creates aroma) makes them excellent candidates for energy medicine investigation.
- Oils possess a much higher frequency than the plants from which they are derived.
- Individual oils may be blended to enhance effects, but this requires considerable experience as an aromatherapist.
- Oils may be inhaled, defused, ingested, or applied topically. Specified oils require specialized application.
- Oils are widely used in mainstream medicine in Europe.

Chapter Seven

Energy Medicine

There is a body of knowledge within the alternative movement that has been growing tremendously in popularity. It is the result of a new understanding of the nature of reality. Some writers refer to it as "energy medicine," others as "vibrational medicine," and still others as "frequency medicine." They are all referring to the same thing. Arbitrarily, and not because any one label is superior to another, I choose to use the term "energy medicine" throughout this discussion.

The origins of energy medicine are hinted at in many ancient cultures, although a scientific understanding of the underlying principles was in all probability lacking. From ancient times there has been an almost universal belief that there was some "vital force,' or energy, or spirit that was at the fundamental core of human body existence and its healing mechanisms. This belief held sway in the western world up to the era in which scientific biomedicine began to dominate, and began to think of the human body as a machine and the mind as a biochemical electrical process, and not as a universal and integrative life force. In the Eastern world the concept of life force would survive to the present day as chi, prana, or chakra. In the arena of modern alternative medicine, energy medicine provides scientific foundation for many of these ancient beliefs, and also takes on many other forms (which will be detailed shortly). Modern conventional medicine tends to lump all energy medicine under the term "vitalism," a term once used to describe underlying life force, but which is a term that conveys a very negative connotation as it is being understood by its modern biomedical detractors.

Throughout this book we have made references to the new understanding of reality as evidenced by the discoveries of quantum physics. It is now time to revisit that discipline in greater detail. Modern medicine claims that its legitimacy rests on scientific validation, and, to an extent, this is true. But the science of modern medicine is the science of Isaac Newton's mechanistically conceived universe, which modern medicine only succeeded in emulating roughly three hundred years after Newton discovered his laws. Newton conceived of a universe that was absolutely predictable, ruled by knowable laws. The human body was viewed as a machine, and modern medicine concurs.

Newton's scientific methodology called for breaking things down into their elemental components, a process referred to as scientific reductionism, as the manner in which laws would be discovered. Science has continued to pursue this approach to the present day. The pursuit has led science into the quantum world, a flexible, plastic, non–predictable world, wherein the laws of the Newtonian world simply do not apply. Science has evolved far beyond the mechanistic view and seeks new understanding of the nature of reality. Modern medicine, in large measure, remains locked in the mechanistic view.

Quantum physics has proven that matter is nothing more than highly concentrated energy. Most of what appears to be solid is actually space, held together by a force similar to gravity. The solid objects that we think we see are actually illusion. Following the line of thinking of quantum physics, the human body is not a machine; it is, in a very real sense, a concentrated energy pattern, that continually interacts with the energy "soup" within which it swims.

The human body is possessed of no fixed boundaries. As humans we are constantly shedding electrons and picking up new ones. A room full of people are literally exchanging energy bits, with each other and with their environment. There is a constantly changing malleable process taking place. The reason we continue to be identifiable is due to the fact that the energy pattern that we are is an integrated energy pattern. Necessarily, viewing the human body as concentrated energy rather than as machine, suggests profound implications for interpreting disease, and even reality. It offers a very different paradigm than the mechanism of Isaac Newton provides. Modern scientific medicine has a difficult time accepting where science is leading.

The law of entropy holds that order leads to disorder, integration to disintegration, and concentration to dilution. Every cell in the human body is replaced within seven years, the cells of some organs replacing themselves much more rapidly. Yet our outward appearance remains relatively unchanged. Even with advanced age our essential features are still recognizable. Some force is holding us together. Similarly, astrophysicists speak of "dark matter," or negative entropy. Some unknown force or anti magnetic property is causing the universe to expand at an increasing rate, yet the known laws of gravity and Big Bang theory state that the universe should be slowing in its expansion. What is it?

Energy reality is viewed as conscious reality; the universe is viewed as intelligent. These beliefs, held by allegedly primitive societies, are continually belittled. Yet highly educated researchers, trained in the methodology of science, are now validating them. If we think of the human brain as a biological computer, and various emotions and feelings as resulting from chemical or hormonal factors, we are interpreting reality from the mechanistic science paradigm. Yet if we think of the brain as the link with the conscious universe, and emotions and feelings as energy patterns, we are of the quantum paradigm.

In the quantum world things believed absurd in the mechanical world are commonplace reality. If we accept the belief of quantum physics that every particle of the universe, no matter how minute, contains within itself the entire universe, our thinking most assuredly must change. Healing would then become an issue of tapping in to the universal source, and the energy field that comprises the human body, interacting with the conscious universe in a manner totally unfathomable to conventional medicine. Modern quantum physicists refer to this concept of reality as "self aware" universe, holographic universe, energy universe, intelligent universe, etc. These are the terms being used by highly educated exponents of the scientific approach. Science is leading scientists to accept an entirely new concept of reality. Science is leading them to an entirely new way of viewing the human body and of promoting its healing processes.

Some of the new paradigm has found its way into conventional medicine. Geneticists and molecular biologists certainly utilize some of the discoveries of reductionistic science, but they are still locked in on the mechanical fix: find the defective gene, hormone, or enzyme, and the problem will be solved. The mechanical fix mentality continues to exist; what needs to be fixed has simply gotten smaller. The concept of there being physical causes for all disease that necessitates a physical cure continues to exist. In fairness, it should be noted that within the mindset, but limited by it, some notable achievements have been attained.

Conventional physicians are beginning to recognize the mind–spirit–body connection. Unfortunately, this connection is recognized only within the context of emotions, and the response is to control emotions with psychosomatic medicine. Conventional medicine has thus far remained unable to make the transition to the new scientific paradigm.

Some forms of energy healing are very old, and have been traditionally disparaged, while many others are relatively new, fueled by scientific advances. In this chapter we shall review both old and new as they represent the new science of energy medicine.

The new energy medicine adds the dimension of the non–physical, of consciousness, to the healing process. Within the scope of the empirically known physical world, mechanical responses possess validity. But this validity is limited. If the emotional state of an individual can bring about illness or aid in promoting healing, is it not also a causative factor in the maintenance of health?

Thinkers have long concerned themselves with what happens to the "person" when the physical body dies. According to the mechanistic view it also dies. In the energy view the "spirit" is what had temporarily occupied the body, and when the body dies the spirit goes on. There is a spiritual dimension to energy medicine. Quantum physicists are reuniting science with the theology and philosophy that earlier scientists managed to disassociate when they secularized reality. The energy approach is a more integrated and global approach. More than just a body, human beings have been devalued by the mechanistic approach.

Some forms of energy are accepted by conventional medicine: the chemical energy of the digestive process, also known as metabolic energy, and the electrical energy used by the brain, some organs, and the nervous system. Modern medicine has also discovered that cells communicate with each other with bursts of ultra violet light. Various forms of communication are constantly taking place within the body. Communication implies intelligence. Conventional medicine recognizes and accepts these energy systems, but it is not willing to go beyond them, to more subtle levels of energy and their implications.

Other types of energy are generally accepted. Geopathic energy is earth energy: earth poles, plate tectonics, vortices, ley lines, etc. Electromagnetic energy is that which results from cell phones, radio waves, television beams, and electrical transmission. Additionally, various types of energy radiates from the sun; most of the more harmful rays are deflected away. We are living in an energy soup.

Eastern Energy Beliefs

Traditional Chinese medicine believes in the existence of chi, or life force. Some chi is inherited, some chi is constantly being replenished through nutrition, and some chi is absorbed from the environment through specific points in the body. These body absorption points are the acupuncture points. Traditional Chinese medicine has held for thousands of years that it is the interrupting or blocking of these points along the body's energy grid (meridians) that causes disease.

The Hindu tradition contributes the chakras, or, seven major energy and emotional centers in the body. Each chakra is believed to be associated with a particular region of the body, a certain gland, certain nerves, and specific emotional issues. The five lower chakras are associated with emotions. The sixth chakra is associated with intellectual issues, while the seventh chakra is concerned with spiritual issues. Some claim there is an eighth chakra located outside of and above the body that serves as a link through which the infinite spiritual joins with the seventh chakra. The interconnectedness of a variety of associations in each chakra suggests that there are much more complicated issues in healing than mechanistic scientific medicine would allow.

The physical body is subject to the laws of the physical world at its level of existence. Purely physical needs require physical responses. But the energy body that surrounds and influences the physical body responds to different stimuli. Yoga, in its various forms, is believed to maintain the chakras. T'ai chi and its close relative chi gong, concern themselves with the movement of chi energy along the meridian system of the physical body. These techniques emphasize slow, graceful movement and breathing exercises to move and recharge the chi. Yoga and t'ai chi, in all their derivations, are energy activities.

Energy and Religious Beliefs

In addition to chi and chakra, there are various ethereal energies believed to surround the physical body. These energies take a variety of forms, and many are associated with religious beliefs. There is an ancient belief that the physical body is enveloped in layers of energy bodies, each layer manifesting a higher and higher frequency as it distances itself from the physical body. Some spiritualists see this layering as the way in which spirit manifests itself in physicality: the gradual gearing down of frequency until it reaches the level of dense matter. This process is also believed to be the avenue through which individuals reconnect with their spiritual origins. Many who channel entities through themselves credit their ability to being able to raise their vibrational level to allow the event to occur.

In Christian belief the concept of the Trinity has been explained as the gearing down of infinite vibration in the Mind of God to the Christ Consciousness, and eventually, to the Holy Spirit, through which direct connection can be made. A similar mechanism for contact with the Source is found in the Hindu Trinity of Brahman, Visnu, and Shiva. Similarly, the sound of Om is considered to be the vibration of physicality, of the Holy Spirit or of Shiva made manifest, and is chanted in religious cloisters throughout the world. The sound of Om is the sound of creation.

Religious traditions abound with ethereal beings. Whether they are the various brotherhoods of light beings found within the teachings of the Saint Germain Society, the ascended masters concept of George Gurdjieff (The Fourth Way), angels or avatars, humanity believes, and has always believed, in a non–physical dimension of reality. Even the popular television science fiction series *Star Trek* portrayed the character "Q," an entity that could materialize anywhere, anytime, in any form, and who resided with other like beings in the "continuum." The worlds of science, theology, and the paranormal, all merge in belief systems that embrace ethereal beings

Proof that an ethereal body, or energy field, surrounds the human body is provided by kirlian photography, a process that is able to project the aura, or energy field, on to a photosensitive plate. Sometimes seeing is believing. A number of years ago, while traveling across the country, I stopped to visit a cousin in Hot Springs, Arkansas. He is a chiropractor by profession, uses crystals in his therapy, and has built a kirlian photography apparatus. To demonstrate he photographed my right hand; the resultant aura was visible but quite weak. He suggested that this was due to my rather low energy level, to which I readily agreed, as I had driven the entire night to avoid being caught in an ice storm. He changed the subject, began talking about his crystals, and handed me one as a gift. Not knowing what to do with it at the moment, I carried it around with me as we toured his center.

After about thirty minutes had passed he suggested that we photograph my aura again. The aura was much brighter. Thirty minutes later he did it again and the aura was brighter still. He attributed my increased energy field to the "energy collector" I had been holding: the crystal (more on crystals later). I still have in my possession the three sets of photos of my aura, proof that some source of energy surrounds the body.

Within religious tradition angels, saints, and holy persons are depicted with a halo around their heads, indicating their higher vibrational or spiritual level. Visions of celestial beings are usually described as shimmering light beings, transparent but distinguishable, not entirely real, ghostlike. The auras of many authentic spiritual teachers have been observed by their students. Some clairvoyants claim the ability to see and read auras, even to the point of observing thought forms. Clairvoyants also claim the ability to determine a person's physical and emotional state by the colors they observe in their aura. On a less ethereal level, what does an infrared scanner "see?"

The most awesome aspect of kirlian photography is the so–called "phantom effect." Cutting away a part of a leaf and then photographing the remaining leaf reveals the aura of the entire leaf. Physically, part of the leaf has been removed, but on an ethereal level, the energy leaf remains. The phantom effect has also been observed in human subjects who have undergone amputations. How does one account for the presence of the image of something that does not appear to be there?

Health intuitives, clairvoyants, psychics, and those who channel, often posit that their ability stems from the "reading" or the sensing of subtle vibrational levels. There are some who hold to the belief that every thought ever expressed exists eternally in sort of a timeless frequency library, referred to as the Akashic Records. Some psychics claim the ability to tune into the Akashic Records, just as we would tune a station on the radio. The information is always there; to be heard all that is required is a properly tuned receiver. All that was or will be, is. "The flap of a butterfly's wings resonates throughout the universe," is a poetic but appropriate representation of the concept of universal interconnectedness, a concept that seems to explain some of the bizarre results of experiments in quantum physics.

The ancient *Vedas* hold that in the beginning there existed only energy. Some of that energy became conscious. This consciousness was the rishis, who were light or frequency entities who remained apart from physical creation. Ancient Chinese tradition refers to this period as the time of the Void. Some of the conscious energy eventually manifested itself in physicality—the act of creation. The purpose of physicality was to experience and observe, sort of an entertainment. For a great period of time light entities moved back and forth between spirit and matter, but gradually, became addicted to physical sensation.

The moving from the non physical to the physical required a lowering of vibrational level or frequency. Visits to the physical world would last longer and longer until, finally, the light entities became trapped in the physical world. When they became physical they became aware of Self, and this awareness was the split from the Source. *A Course in Miracles* refers to the act of separation as the recognition of self as distinct from its Source, continually splitting until it creates the ultimate act of separation, the illusion of body and the physical world. All the great scriptures of the world contain a version of the splitting away from God by the human race.

The Mind-Body Connection

Many belief systems hold that there are various levels of energy bodies between the Source and the physical body. Generally, the body closest to the physical body is the ethereal, or energy body. This is the body that is witnessed through the medium of kirlian photography. Next is the astral body, which possesses mobility of its own, consciousness, and emotion. It can project its consciousness away from the physical body in what is termed astral projection or out–of–body experience. The next body is the mental body wherein thought forms are said to exist. Ideas or thoughts, it is believed, are creation, and as such, they possess a physical reality (but more of this shortly). Beyond the mental is the causal body, or the area in which the soul resides. This body houses the stored experiences and incarnations of that particular being.

Some of this belief is found within the modern concept of right brain–left brain. The right hemisphere of the brain is creative and artistic. The left hemisphere is logical and quantitative. The right brain pertains to the unconscious self, while the left brain pertains to the conscious self. The right brain uses symbolic language; it dreams and is visual. The left brain uses literal language and is analytical. Some claim that the right brain is the physical part of us that is trying to stay in contact with the Source, and to receive the symbolic communication from It. Right brain thinking is devalued in western society, but so–called primitive cultures seem to have placed far greater importance on right brain issues. Waking dreams, symbolism, and the integration and relationship of various life forces are part of the ancient traditions. However, the literal and logical left brain is what modern society values and rewards.

Thought is the process in mind by which substance is acted on by energy, directed by intelligence. Thought is a frequency and can manifest itself as creative power. Nothing can happen in the objective world unless it is balanced equally in the subjective world. Some clairvoyants claim that thought manifests itself so powerfully that they can see it as thought symbols in surrounding energy bodies. Universally held thought is collective consciousness. When a concept appears in the collective consciousness it immediately exists everywhere, as is evidenced by the Hundred Monkey Story. The sum of the total exists in all its parts. Thought influences the physical.

By way of example, individuals who think optimistically generally possess better immune systems than do pessimistic thinkers, who tend to be sick much more often. Optimistic people tend to attempt control over their lives, while pessimists tend to buy into the cult of victimization. Both types of thinkers tend to associate with their own kind. Pessimists exude a negative energy that drains the energy of those around them, whereas optimists exude a vitalizing and energizing force.

The naysayer in a sales organization is not around very long. People who dwell on past negative experiences will eventually drag down their own bodily energy. If not released this practice generally will manifest itself as ill health. Remembering an event is not the same thing as dwelling on the event. In the progression of life knowledge and understanding should derive from experiencing. Hanging on to traumatic events is not progressing, nor is it concentrating on the present, the now.

Some believe that the planet is encased in millennia of negative thought buildup. All of the wars, the hatred, and the perpetrated injustices are believed to have accumulated in a negative energy field. Astral travelers have claimed to experience nasty little creatures, presumed to be negative incarnations, during their out–of–body projections. Other people believe that any body of thought, whether it is judged good or bad, will eventually manifest itself. This belief would seem to indicate that if thought can manifest, then thought can be used to control and direct the course of our lives.

Herein is derived a large body of practice and belief. One of the oldest and most consistently held beliefs is the belief in the power of prayer. True prayer is not asking for specific things or happenings; it is asking for nothing. It is quieting the mind, and attempting to reconnect with the Source. Prayer does not necessarily consist of the uttering of memorized passages, chanting, or reciting in staccato (although there is validity in these practices); it may be silence. Emptying the mind, meditating, is prayer.

In a sense prayer is affirmation. The use of affirmation is a strategy that is widely taught by self–improvement gurus today. The trick lies in the wording of the affirmation. Think carefully about what it is that you desire and the ramifications of obtaining it, because you just might receive literally what you sought. Another strategy involves visualization, seeing oneself in a certain situation, or performing a particular action or physical movement repeatedly in one's mind, and feeling it. Many athletes have used these techniques quite successfully to improve their performance. All of these activities are energy exercises.

It is widely held that human beings are more than purely physical beings; they are multidimensional. Disturbances or imbalances in any of their energy bodies can translate itself into the physical as an illness. It also suggests that the treatment of illness involves more than a physical treatment. Further, perhaps the only true healing results from what we hold within our multidimensional selves.

It is hoped that this general introduction to the concept of living, interactive energy will aid the reader in gaining a greater appreciation of the energy medicine modalities that we are now going to consider.

Acupuncture

Perhaps the oldest and best known form of energy medicine is acupuncture. The first references to acupuncture as a Chinese medical treatment date back five thousand years. Acupuncture involves placing needles in to acupoints, or entry points, in the body's meridian system. Traditional Chinese medicine holds that the body contains established energy pathways, meridians, and the strategic placement of needles along meridian acupoints restores balance, removes blockages, and improves health. Traditional Chinese physicians use acupuncture to treat all manner of diseases, human and animal. In most instances the treatment appears to exert positive influences on health.

Western medical researchers have tried all sorts of ways to evaluate and determine the underlying principles of acupuncture—with little success. What has been validated is that acupoints display a measurably lower electrical resistance than does surrounding tissue. There has also been a number of investigations utilizing sophisticated scientific techniques, that indicate that there are flow points in the body that reflect ancient meridian charts, both for humans and for animals.

We might think of the meridian system as a network of tubes, an energy pipeline traversing the body, and acupoints as control valves in the pipeline. Acupuncture either increases or decreases the energy flow to restore proper balance. It is now a proven fact that the body does possess a meridian system and it does possess acupoints. How they work remains an unsolved mystery.

Traditional Chinese medicine combines acupuncture with its belief in five elemental energies: wood, fire, earth, metal, and water. Wood is associated with the liver and gall bladder and the sour taste. Fire is associated with the small intestine, sex organs, and heart and the bitter taste. Earth is associated with the spleen, pancreas, and stomach and the sweet taste. Metal is associated with the lungs and the large intestine and the spicy taste. There appears to be a more demonstrable association regarding water, for it is associated with the bladder and kidney and the salty taste. There are a number of other characteristics associated with each of the five elemental energies, and various elaborate charts indicate their interrelationships. Entire books have been written on the subject.

The bottoms of the feet, the hands, and the ears, are considered specialties of acupuncture. View a reflexology chart to obtain some insight into this system. It is believed that different regions of the foot, hand, and ear, correspond to different regions or organs of the body. In some instances this has been proven to be scientifically correct. Specific areas of the body are believed to replicate the entire body. Part of traditional Chinese acupuncture involves using whole body acupuncture in conjunction with one or more specific area acupunctures. Interestingly, the leaf of a tree is a miniature representation of the structure of the entire tree.

Acupuncture has been used successfully in treating various types of pain. In China it is used as a drugless anesthetic. The success rate of pain management by acupuncture in the United States is significant, but not as high as it is claimed to be in China. Whether this difference is due to the skill level of the practitioner, cultural acceptance, or reporting technique, is begging the question. The results are noteworthy.

Mainstream American medicine is beginning to incorporate acupuncture. It has been found to be particularly effective in treating victims of stroke and neurological damage. It appears to aid in restoring or rerouting neural pathways much quicker and more thoroughly than conventional physical therapy and drugs, especially when used in conjunction with physical therapy. The treatment of choice for these conditions in China is acupuncture alone. In China acupuncture has been used to treat practically every known disease, claiming moderate to substantial success. Experience with widespread treatment use in the West is either quite limited or non–existent. Acupuncture has been used, with quite impressive results, in the treatment of drug, alcohol, and tobacco addiction, in both the United Kingdom and the United States.

The trend in the United States is away from the use of needles in acupuncture. In their place an electric stimulator pulses charges at acupoints, in what is believed to be a safer, more efficient technique. Some traditional acupuncturists enhance their procedures by using a process known as moxibustion. The handle of each needle is wrapped with the mugwort herb, which is then ignited. Heat from the burning mugwort, or mox, is transferred down through the inserted needle to enhance its effect. Some practitioners use acupressure to achieve similar effects. Various other energy devices are also used and will be outlined as different energy treatments are described.

Acupuncture is moving into mainstream medicine in the United States. A number of allopathic physicians, especially those specializing in geriatrics, have obtained training of the treatment and use it in their practices. Naturopaths and some chiropractors use various forms of acupuncture, as do some physical therapists. It goes without stating that those who practice traditional Chinese medicine use it extensively.

Magnet Therapy

Magnets, or more correctly, magnetic properties, have been known to exist for several thousand years. The often repeated legend of a ancient Greek shepherd named Magnus, being attracted to a large lodestone, has many derivations: the iron nails in his sandals, or the metallic tip of his cane (or staff), were attracted to the rock. In any event the term magnet derives from the hero of the legend.

Magnets were used in healing in ancient times. More accurately, pieces of magnetic rock were used, in that artificial magnets did not appear until the 1820's. Ancient Greek, Indian, Egyptian, and Chinese texts make mention of various healing effects claimed for the use of magnets.

By the first century of the modern era the Chinese were using a magnetic compass. A thousand years later Viking and Arab seamen adapted it to ocean going navigation. In the late eighteenth century a German physician, Franz Anton Mesmer, popularized magnetic healing. Mesmer claimed that humans possessed an "animal magnetism," and it was irregular patterns in this magnetism that caused illness. Strategic placement of magnets upon the body would restore or rebalance the body's subtle magnetic field. On occasion Mesmer would forego the magnets and use his hands only to achieve the same results (see below).

Paracelsus, Samuel Hahnemann, and Louis Pasteur, all believed in the healing power of magnets. During the nineteenth century magnets were widely advertised as the ultimate panacea to cure practically every ailment. Ironically it was a Chicago pitchman, J. C. Thacher, founder of the Chicago Magnet Company, who claimed that the placing of magnets in the shoes and the clothes, would move energy throughout the body by influencing iron in the blood. It was not until 1954 when Linus Pauling discovered the magnetic properties of hemoglobin, that some scientific basis for the earlier claim was advanced.

Human beings evolved on a planet replete with geomagnetic forces and are adapted to their environment. Obviously, the altering of the environment would have ramifications for the human species. During the early days of the space program, although an artificial environment conductive to sustaining life was provided for astronauts, health problems were still being experienced. What was not being provided was an artificial magnetic field to mimic the one left back on the planet's surface. Today space suits contain magnets and spacecraft contain magnetic field generators.

Apparently, ancient peoples were much more attuned to a need to relate to earth energy than are modern day humans. Ancient structures, particularly religious ones, were built upon lines of geomagnetic concentration. The uplifting effect that can be achieved by visiting an old church may partly be due to the geomagnetic forces of its location. Ancient peoples held places to be holy perhaps due to the higher frequencies that were being experienced at those sites. The concept of "dwelling place of the gods" may have some explanation in a study of ley lines or vortices.

There is growing evidence to suggest that modern steel girded buildings shield out much of the earth's natural energy necessary for optimum health. In pre industrial society the cells of the human body and the frequency of the earth's magnetic field, resonated at the same frequency, 7.8 cycles per second. There was harmony; there was balance. In the modern world, technology has bombarded the planet with additional frequencies, the bulk of which come from communications devices and electrical transmission lines. But most modern kitchens contain a microwave oven, and microwaves "kill" the food whose molecules they agitate. What is the long–range effect for human health?

A number of bodily processes are electrically charged, and are therefore subject to magnetic influences. What role that magnets might play in creating either positive or negative effects is being researched. Some of the research indicates that magnets can help some conditions and worsen others. It seems to depend on which polarity to use for which condition.

Is the body's reaction to subtle magnetic energy forces what ancient people referred to as vitalism? Will modern science eventually "prove" what ancients already "knew?" Is the law of attraction just a saying, or, are individuals literally physically (or energetically) attracted to each other. When a person develops "bad vibes" is this just an expression, or is it the recognition on some subtle level of disharmonious frequency? The human body is an energy generator. It is a proven scientific fact that "healing hands" generate a measurable magnetic field.

Studies conducted in a number of different countries indicate positive effects of magnetic therapy in reducing pain. Studies in the former Soviet Union suggested that magnet therapy was effective in treating cancers without surgery and chemotherapy. Magnet therapy is not an FDA approved treatment in the United States, so major research monies are not forthcoming. Nonetheless, the eventually positive use of magnet therapy is a tantalizing subject.

Light Therapy

Merely introducing the concept that light might be considered a healing modality generally evokes a negative response. Yet light heals and is used in mainstream medicine. Light is frequency, and therefore, is a form of energy medicine. Consider the role of sunlight in the production of vitamin D. Consider the role of light (or the lack of light) in the production of melatonin (in darkness) and seratonin (in light). Light plays a major role in the natural rhythm of the body, the circadian rhythm cycle. Light deprivation has led to the labeling of its effects as Seasonal Affective Disorder, usually affecting people during the winter months, when daylight is limited, but significantly affecting people living in the far North, where daylight is absent during the winter months, and swing shift workers, whose biological clocks are in constant turmoil. Cycles of light and dark are a part of the environment in which we evolved and affect how we function.

Color consists of different frequencies within the light spectrum. It has long been known by psychologists and other therapists, that color affects mood. Certain colors, those at the high end of light frequency, red, orange, and yellow, are stimulating. Colors of lower frequency, green, blue, and violet, produce a sedative or calming effect. There is ongoing research on the use of different colored lights and their effect on acupoints, again, emphasizing that different colors are different frequencies. Energy bodies have been linked with certain colors of the light spectrum. Different colors have been attributed to different chakras. Colored light, it seems, has always played a role in subtle energy thinking.

Light therapy is more widely accepted than many people realize. Surgical lasers are being produced to emit a specific color of light; certain color lasers are more effective for certain types of procedures. One form of high technology, photodynamic therapy, consists of injecting certain types of light sensitive dyes into the body. In some cases these dyes are used to diagnose; in others, specific light activated dyes will bind with cancer cells and kill them when activated. Part of the ultra violet frequency band is effective for the successful treatment of certain skin disorders and even for some cardiovascular conditions,

Red LED's (light emitting diodes) are widely used in Europe as a standard mainstream treatment modality. Pulsing red LED's have been used for a variety of brain wave activities. The steady beam has been used in lieu of needles on acupoints and to promote the healing of injured tissue.

Some literature suggests that the red LED maintains the same frequency as a healthy cell, and promotes healing through the principle of resonance. The principle of resonance holds that nature seeks harmony, and if left to its own devices, will achieve homeostasis. Resonance can also be described by quoting the well known expression: "two hearts beat as one."

Subtle Energy Healing Approaches

Experience seems to indicate that the various energy approaches thus mentioned do not work the same for all who use them. It seems that intuitives, clairvoyants, mystics, and psychics, are much more successful than other individuals. This suggests that some people may be more attuned to subtle energy forces than others are. It further suggests that the ancient concepts of "the laying on of hands," remote healing, and the like, are not without some foundation.

Do some individuals possess the power to focus healing energy? Controlled laboratory studies indicate that this is so, and further indicate that this type of healing has an effect similar to magnetic healing. The earliest verification of the power of healers came from studying the efforts of "born" natural healers, primarily working with plants and animals to avoid subtle personality issues. Dr. Dolores Krieger worked with human patients and also non natural healers, her premise being that just about everyone possesses the innate power to focus energy and promote healing. So she developed and taught energy focusing techniques, the ultimate result being the development of a system known as Therapeutic Touch, an approach which is infiltrating mainstream medicine.

Causes for hands–on–healing powers have been attributed to energy exchange (empathy), the channeling of divine energy (prayer), and bioinformational exchange or geomagnetic restructuring (resonance) at the ethereal level. Resonance seems to be a key factor. Somehow the proper frequencies for the promotion of healing are transferred to the body of the patient by the healer. Hands–on–healing, sometimes referred to as bioenergetic healing, is an integral part of mainstream medicine in many parts of the world, the one great bastion of resistance being the United States.

A form of energy healing that is growing in popularity in the United States is Reiki. The Japanese, Mikao Usui, developed the technique approximately a century ago, basing his system on a study and amalgamation of the teachings of Jesus and Buddha. Reiki channels healing energy into the body through the hands, preceded by the drawing of specific symbols in the air with the hands to amplify the healing force. Reiki employs no force and no pressure; energy is simply allowed to flow. Advanced Reiki practitioners (there are three levels of Reiki training) can activate energy flow with parts of their body other than the hands. Traditionally, the symbols used in the various levels of Reiki were to be reserved only for those who had undergone the appropriate attunement, but recently, texts written for popular consumption have appeared with diagrams of the symbols.

Arising out of the Hindu tradition, pranic healing is similar to acupuncture in that it involves moving energy around the chakras of the patient, the significant difference being that the hands are used instead of needles. Pranic healing utilizes breathing techniques and visualization exercises as part of the process. Pranic healers claim positive results for a large variety of medical problems. A unique aspect of pranic healing involves the ability to heal at a distance, placing the method somewhat within the camp of spiritual healing.

The subtle nature of energy healing has produced many skeptics. Scientifically controlled experiments, however, indicate positive effects from energy healing. Some have attributed this to placebo effect, but if one chooses to push the holographic model of the universe to its extreme conclusions, everything is placebo effect, because everything emanates from universal idea. Successful results with energy healing of plants and animals would tend to weaken the placebo effect argument.

Water as Energy Healer

The belief and use of water as an energy healing agent is of ancient origins. The healing powers of water are recognized throughout the scriptural traditions of the world. NASA's search for water, for where there is water there can be life, is valid in more ways than one. Healing powers have been attributed to various waters worldwide, some grounded in mineral springs, others in religious belief systems. Franklin Roosevelt's famous hot mineral baths and the healing powers of Lourdes are but two famous examples.

Life evolved from the sea, and there remains a fascination with the beach, the lake, and the mountain stream. The widespread presence of spas, hot tubs, swimming pools, and fountains, are indicators of the power of and interest in water. Various forms of hydrotherapy have been used in physical therapy for some time. Birthing tubs are being used, although not generally, to ease the discomfort of natural childbirth. Relaxing in a treated hot bath and the stimulation of the Swedish cold plunge reflect both physical and emotional responses from water.

The nineteenth century German water cure movement crossed to America where it manifested itself in the health spa movement and provided the foundation for the development of naturopathy. It was hardly the first water cure movement in Europe. European history from the middle ages forward is replete with such movements. For the better part of the twentieth century the unique characteristics of magnetized water have been known. The introduction of catalyst altered water by John Willard was but a beginning.

Water, it seems, possesses some rather unique characteristics. It is proven to be an excellent storage medium for various subtle energies, and since ninety percent of all the molecules in the human body are water molecules, the potential ramifications of just this one characteristic are considerable. Water can function as a memory system capable of storing information. Water molecules can be made to cluster, providing greater and quicker movement through the body. Water can also be altered to become the vehicle for carrying micro nutrients through the body. Water can be made wetter; it can be altered to absorb free radicals.

Recent research suggests that water "remembers" what was in it, and reacts to positive and negative emotions. Substances in water apparently can be serially diluted, as in homeopathy, yet their ability to function remains as if they were physically present. Water can be patterned and water can be imprinted. Water appears capable of being altered remotely. Possibilities are endless but many seem to fall within the more esoteric field of radionics.

Radionics

Radionics is a modality that utilizes various devices and instruments to detect, diagnose, and provide therapy at the energy level. Radionics enthusiasts believe that instruments can be constructed (and have already been constructed) that can sense and amplify what is going on in the body at an energy level, without ever actually touching the body, and can treat conditions in exactly the same manner. The reputed founder of radionics is Dr. Albert Abrams, a nineteenth century San Francisco based neurologist.

Every disease has a specific frequency (also applicable to essential oils as discussed in the last chapter). It is detectable in the body or in a speck of blood or tissue from that body. Through an elaborate testing process Abrams identified many different diseases by the amount of energy they emitted, measured in ohms. His complicated diagnostic process involved a measuring device, a healthy surrogate (human subject), a drop of blood from the diseased patient, and hard wired connections between the three components. Incidentally, the process would not work unless the human surrogate was lined up on magnetic west. How this worked remains a mystery, but Abrams is credited with building the world's first radionic measuring instrument.

Radionics is based on a belief that everything generates a subtle energy field that can be psychically sensed by properly attuned individuals. Radionic instruments apparently can pick up this subtle energy reading without the aid of a health intuitive.

Building on the work of Abrams was a chiropractor, Ruth Drown, who claimed that the treating of a diagnosed blood spot of a patient cured the patient. Some sort of resonance factor appeared to connect patient and patient specimen, even at considerable distance. Interestingly, an experiment in quantum physics involves the splitting of a proton so that its two halves were traveling away from each other, each at the speed of light. When one half of the proton was made to make an abrupt turn, simultaneously so did the other half, with no observable connection between the two halves, and in apparent violation of the alleged ultimate speed limit of light speed. This experiment could lend credence to the validity of remote or distance healing.

Some radionics experimenters reputedly use photographs of the individuals, animals, or plants being treated to create a cure. Two twentieth century individuals, working independently of each other, used this technique to treat plant diseases: Curtis Upton and T. Galen Hieronymous. Supposedly, they concentrated on plants to lessen the controversy of such treatment claims, and to minimize the scrutiny of the medical establishment.

Experiments in the United Kingdom led to the development of imprinting. Vials filled with fluid or small bottles of plain tablets were imprinted with the vibrational pattern of a known remedy through the use of a radionic device known as the Rae Potency Stimulator. Radionics practitioners claim they can duplicate any vibrational or homeopathic remedy in any potency by using this device.

Magnetism seems to play a role in imprinting, just as it does in the duplicating, or imprinting, of blank cassette tapes when copying an original. Rae also developed geometric shapes to reflect specific remedies. He did this by dowsing the outline or "shape" of a remedy. This sounds quite far fetched, but scientific experiments have proven that sounds generate specific geometric patterns. Grains of sand placed on a smooth surface will rearrange themselves into a precise geometric pattern when under the influence of specific pitches (frequencies).

One of the biggest names in the frequency medicine field is that of Raymond Royal Rife (mentioned in the preceding chapter). His invention of a super resolution microscope during the 1920's catapulted him to national and international fame. He later observed living organisms through his microscope, and by experimenting with frequencies, and by observing the effects of these frequencies on various organisms, he gradually identified a number of disease killing frequencies. Inasmuch as the march of scientific medicine was well underway, reaction to Rife's claims met with ridicule, resistance, criticism, and disbelief..

In 1934 an experiment was arranged at the University of Southern California that involved a team of medical doctors and sixteen terminally ill cancer patients. Rife's frequency treatments reputedly cured all sixteen patients. What then followed was a string of disastrous events, providing tantalizing tidbits for conspiracy theory advocates.

Rife's laboratory was broken into, equipment vandalized, and records removed (copies kept at other sites survived). The supportive head of the Southern California chapter of the AMA suddenly died, just hours before a scheduled press conference announcing the results of the USC experiment. It has been claimed that data later indicated that he died from arsenic laced toothpaste. A New Jersey laboratory working on the Rife project burned down mysteriously in the middle of the night. The AMA, after its president Morris Fishbien had unsuccessfully attempted to buy into Rife's company (1938), became a vitriolic foe of his approach. Needless to state, the pharmaceutical industry and the FDA made common cause in their opposition as well. The legacy of Raymond Rife appeared to be lost.

Rife had claimed that his invention provided a drugless, non–invasive, inexpensive, and side effect free treatment procedure that was effective in treating a number of diseases. Litigation, financial pressures, and wide-spread discrediting by many of his former supporters, allowed his work to languish. But some Rife supporters, working with various notes and records that survived, have reconstructed much of his research, and as of this writing, a number of companies sell frequency generating machines which they claim are based on Rife's discoveries. These devices are not available for medical treatment, nor have they been evaluated or approved by the medical establishment. They may be purchased and used only for personal experimentation, and evidence of their efficacy is largely anec-dotal. Health professionals are not allowed to own Rife devices; as a result, professional investigation of their merits cannot be undertaken.

In light of discoveries in quantum physics and the subsequent new understanding of reality, there is strong evidence to suggest that frequency, or energy medicine, may very well be the wave of the future. A concen-trated focused light has created a new and more precise and bloodless form of surgery, while concentrated focused sound is being used successfully in prostate cancer treatment, and research is underway to remove fibroid tumors with the same technique. The problem is not with the new tech-nology; the problem is with the unwillingness of the status quo to accept the magnitude and direction of change resulting from the new quantum science.

Support for Rife's original theories comes from a different, more con-temporary source. Tainio Technologies has developed a device known as a Calibrated Frequency Monitor that measures a range of bioelectrical fre-quencies. Frequencies are measured in units called a hertz. A hertz is one oscillation per second. A kilohertz is 1000 oscillations per second. A megahertz is 1,000,000 oscillations per second. The human body, its organs, natural foods, and all essential oils, are in the hertz range.

A healthy human body oscillates in the range of 62–68 hertz, with the head somewhat higher, except during the sleep state. Interestingly, when body frequency drops below 62 hertz, cells begin to mutate and various diseases begin to appear. The ingesting of "dead" foods lowers the frequency of the body temporarily, thus rendering it more susceptible to disease. The frequency of most foods is in the range from 0 hertz (canned and frozen foods) to 30 hertz (fresh herbs).

The Rife approach called for the use of an instrument capable of generating a frequency which would then be directed toward the body. The theory was that bombarding the body with specific higher frequencies would result in the cure of specific maladies.

Subtle energies do exist, but how radionics works is not known. Some categorically claim that radionics does not work. Perhaps the best possible explanation today is provided by the holographic paradigm. Holograms are created by intersecting two light images of an object in order to create what is referred to as an interference pattern. Imagine two pebbles dropped into still water at some small distance from each other. The ripples of each will expand until they overlap each other. This is an interference pattern. Quantum physicists believe that activity at the quantum level consists of interference patterns, which could lead to the conclusion that the entire universe is a holographic projection. Michael Talbot, in his work *The Holographic Universe,* puts forth this view.

One of the fundamental and bizarre characteristics of a true holographic image, is that if you cut an image in half, each half will contain a projection of the entire image, again, and again, and again, but with each cut being fuzzier than the preceding one. The part does contain the whole. Every aspect of creation, in effect, contains within itself the whole of creation. This phenomenon could explain some of the results of radionics, and if the universe is, indeed, one giant hologram, instantaneous communication within it is a distinct possibility. Perhaps we need huge radionics machines instead of rockets to traverse the universe.

The use of radionics in conventional medicine in the United States is an absolute taboo, the ban sanctioned by both AMA and FDA. At the time of this writing, various devices can be used privately for purposes of personal experimentation and information only.

Chapter Summary

- The conventional medical model is based on a mechanistic universe, yet discoveries in quantum physics are disputing that view.
- All matter is concentrated energy field, interacting with an energy field environment.
- Energy medicine embraces the new physics and incorporates the non- physical dimension into the healing process.
- Ancient cultures believed in universal energy forces: Chinese chi and Hindu chakra for example.
- A belief common to many traditions is that the physical body is surrounded by many layers of non-physical bodies.
- Tradition holds that ethereal bodies of high vibration exist. The halo depicted around the head of saints or the aura some observe emanating from spiritually advanced teachers are examples.
- Kirlian photography provides evidence that energy body exists.
- Sensitives, intuitives, and clairvoyants claim to "sense" or "read" information at the vibrational level.
- Thought is frequency, a process of mind by which substance is acted upon by energy, directed by intelligence.
- Pessimists emit negative energy; optimists exude positive energy. Listening to one's "vibs" has merit.
- The power of prayer, or of creative visualization, is provable quantitatively.
- Humans are multi dimensional beings, consisting of an interconnectedness of body, mind, and spirit.

- One of the oldest forms of energy medicine is acupuncture. The belief is that ill health is the result of blocked energy channels (meridians).
- The efficacy of acupuncture has been proven by modern medicine for the treatment of some conditions.
- Early magnet therapy was viewed as fraud, but science is proving that certain magnetic forces are necessary for the maintenance of health.
- Studies in countries other than the United States indicate positive results being achieved from magnet therapy.
- Periods of light and darkness are necessary for the normal rhythmic functions of the body.
- Colors are different frequencies of the light spectrum and are known to affect mood.
- Surgical lasers utilize light therapy; different color lasers are used for different procedures.
- Photodynamic therapy, utilizing light sensitive dyes, is being used in diagnosis and shows promise for some cancer treatment.
- Red LED's are widely used in Europe to promote healing. They are based on the principle of resonance.
- The "laying on of hands" is an old tradition; Therapeutic Touch is a modern application.
- A number of healing traditions are based on moving or concentrating energy. Reiki and pranic breathing are but two examples.
- The healing power of water has been claimed since ancient times, often within the context of a religious belief system.
- Hydrotherapy is a modern healing modality that employs water.
- Research into the characteristics of water suggests that water remembers, can store information, can be patterned, can be imprinted, and can be clustered.

- Radionics is a modality that uses instruments to promote healing at the energy level.
- Radionics is based on frequency. If a frequency can be determined it can be manipulated.
- Everything that exists has a specific frequency. The belief is that if the frequency of a disease can be determined, it can be altered and the disease can be cured.
- Modern science is able to determine frequencies, and some frequency medicine has found its way into conventional medicine.
- Quantum physics provides credibility for concepts once held to be bizarre.

Chapter Eight

Contemporary Medicine

Contemporary medicine is a contradiction. On the one hand there are many dedicated health care professionals who truly want to serve humanity. Correspondingly, advances in technology have resulted in an almost daily introduction of new lifesaving surgical procedures, intricate medical devices, and powerful pharmaceuticals. In the practice of trauma medicine the United States stands unchallenged. Most certainly, modern medicine has saved or prolonged countless lives. This did not come about without a price.

So on the other hand, modern medicine is viewed as being monopolistic, inordinately expensive, politically dominating, highly institutionalized, commercialized, and impersonal. It has become big business and consumes fifteen percent of the gross national product. More than 4.5 million people earn their living in the health care industry, and this figure represents five percent of the total work force. Only 377,000 of these individuals are medical doctors. And although there are many other licensed and degreed health practitioners, the vast bulk of health care workers never see a patient. They are the researchers, the administrative personnel, the mangers, and the technicians, to name a few.

Medicine has managed to position itself in a central role in society. Such questions as "what is your health worth?" or "how do you place a value on one's life," result in an attitude which, when combined with market forces, translate into astronomical costs for modern American health care.

The medico–industrial complex is equally enmeshed in the political arena, wherein special interests, lobbyists, and lavish contributions influence the political agenda. It is a fact that professional special interest groups exercise disproportionate influence on governmental policy, and the vast bulk of such groups are in the medical profession. Meshing the political agenda with the medical agenda results in further institutionalization of the health care system.

As the new millennium begins, a key issue concerns the cost of pharmaceuticals. The issue is not at all being addressed frontally or honestly. The pharmaceutical industry spends more money on pushing its products (television advertising), than on drug development, yet it claims that the high cost of drugs results from development and approval costs. The result is a drug oriented culture that spent $145 billion on prescription drugs in 2000, and untold billions on various over–the–counter products. The industry lays the blame on its bedfellow, the Food and Drug Administration, whose evaluators are often contract employees from the pharmaceutical industry, and the general public buys into the claim without question. It is automatically assumed that medical care and products should be expensive and will continue to rise in cost. Who raises the question: "Why?"

The new administration is looking at the issue of paying for high cost drugs. It is not looking at the issue of actual cost or profits. It is not looking at the issue of whether or not all this druggery is really necessary. The recent House of Representatives approval of the purchasing of exported FDA approved drugs at substantially lower prices on the foreign market, where governments protect their citizens with state imposed price ceilings, is being touted by the FDA as unsafe. Yet these are FDA approved drugs.

Is it about safety or is it about profit? With whose interests is the FDA concerned: the American consumer or the American pharmaceutical industry?

The Citizen as National Resource

The emergence of the modern nation–state brought with it the valuing of its citizens as resources of the state. The modern state became increasingly concerned with the health of its citizens and with social order issues. Therefore, public health issues were emphasized, and the influence of health care professionals in influencing public health policy escalated. In more authoritarian states the government emphasized and sometimes mandated physical fitness programs.

Emergence of the modern nation–state required the legitimatising of the state. It had to be viewed positively. One result is the emergence of the state role of providing health care services. Government formed a partnership with medicine, and both institutions acquired enhanced status. But modern scientific (and often intrusive) medicine did not emphasize the role of prevention in health care. There is even a question raised by some as to whether it even emphasizes health.

As the state began to set public health laws, medical personnel became legitimate enforcers of the state. In some instances individual freedom and/or the right to privacy were curtailed. Conflicts with personal belief systems, particularly religious beliefs, became more common. Freedom of choice diminished as the establishment medical view became entrenched in government. Democracy and diversity may well be part of the battle cry at the opening of the third millennium, but democracy and diversity do not extend to health care issues. A state sponsored monopoly responds with a resounding negative. Modern medicine is elitist driven and it is monolithic.

Physicians increasingly became the paid agents of the state, the insurance company, the arbitration board, and the corporation. Or they became the paid agents of pharmaceutical companies while performing double duty as paid consultants of the FDA. Professional, ethical, and moral conflicts are inevitable in such a system. As medicine gained in legitimacy, and hence, respectability, it also became increasingly commercialized. Private practices, private institutions, and private hospitals mushroomed, spurred on by promises of greater efficiency and service, and promises of increased profits as well. From the stereotyped doctor's black bag, to the well equipped private office, to the high tech medical center, status and costs grew together. The new medicine concentrated on servicing the affluent. The ability to access and receive "good" medicine became a status symbol.

As medical elites wound their way to advisory boards, and became consultants to government, they became aware of a giant untapped medical marketplace: the non–well–to–do. The only problem lay in finding a revenue source to pay for the medical services.

In America it can be said that politicians "buy" public office in the same manner that a business buys business: by advertising its product or service. For the politician the product is the politician. But in addition to campaign spending (advertising), politicians promise to provide services to their constituents. Elect me and I will provide a promised service or benefit. The cost of the service or benefit, of course, ultimately would be assumed by the United States taxpayer. So government began to increasingly underwrite various types of health services, starting with generally non controversial activities such as inoculations. This development further institutionalized and bureaucratized the practice of medicine.

The United Kingdom enacted the National Health Insurance Act in 1911. Initially highly controversial, and strenuously resisted by the prestigious end of the medical profession, the measure was accepted by the rank–and–file health practitioners, who saw security in the guaranteed payment from the state for becoming a "panel" doctor.

One major cause for the growth of state concern over health issues was due to the numerous wars then plaguing the world. These wars were increasingly fought with conscripted troops, who had to pass a basic health exam as a condition for military service. On both sides of the Atlantic failure rates were appallingly high. Late nineteenth century and early twentieth century governments were not overly concerned about the health of factory workers, but the health of troops was of vital concern.

Between the twentieth century world wars European medical delivery, and the role of the state in providing it, was strongly influenced by the "socializing" of medicine in the Soviet Union. Different countries adopted different approaches, but a commonality was evidenced by their acceptance of the role of the state in providing medical care. For example, Germany and England opted for compulsory medical insurance and state run clinics. Payments to health practitioners were rendered by the state. In France patients could select their own physician, pay the physician out of their own pockets, and then be reimbursed by the state.

Government and Health Care in America

Health care in the United States continued to be market driven, as nineteenth century laissez faire economics continued to dominate. The upgrading of the quality of medical training, a result of the implementing of recommendations in the Flexner Report, reduced the number of medical training institutions, and consequently the number of physicians, and raised the costs. But since the United States was experiencing an unparalleled economic boom from the 1890's to the Crash of 1929, many people paid scant attention to rising medical costs. Elective trips to the physicians office became quite commonplace—for routine checkups, for the acquiring of prescriptions for various pharmaceuticals, or for the seeking of "expert" opinion on a variety of medical issues. Faith in the new medical system also resulted in a mushrooming of minor surgical procedures.

Although initially supportive of the concept of compulsory state health insurance at the opening of the twentieth century, the American Medical Association gradually shifted its position and opposed it. In the Red Scare mentality of the post World War I world (anti communist hysteria), the concept was branded as un–American and pro–Soviet. There was no further need to discuss the issue. The AMA would increasingly become a conservative voice for the American medical establishment. In the 1920's it opposed the creation of veterans hospitals, the disbursing of federal funds for maternal and child care, and even group health insurance plans. All these proposals were viewed as socialistic, and therefore, they were bad.

Various programs of Franklin Roosevelt's New Deal legislative agenda contained health care provisions. The AMA criticized them mildly; in that FDR was an extremely popular leader. Further, the depression had wiped out the ability of many previous paying patients to continue to afford health care. And charitable health care was strained beyond its limits. Obviously, something had to be done if the new medical establishment was going to remain in business.

In 1929, Dallas area teachers contracted with Baylor Union Hospital to provide health care at a fixed rate—the first group hospital plan. The American Hospital Association seized upon the concept, creating Blue Cross/Blue Shield. Since these plans were private insurance plans (capitalistic) rather than compulsory government plans (socialistic), the AMA did not resist them. These developments mark the beginning of the age of private health insurance that was destined to dominate the face of American medicine. Private health insurance was commercial and it was not associated with government. Further, the concept was endorsed by the medical establishment.

Moving through the twentieth century hospitals became the keystones of American medicine. Medical education and medical research were blended into these centers of health care delivery. Costs continued to rise as hospitals were entailing costs not directly associated with the treatment of patients. Hospitals became partly subsidized by public and private sources, They had, in effect, become a major player in the creation of institutionalized medicine.

Medicine and Government Amuck

The mid twentieth century brought the world to a critical juncture. Government had been moving in the direction of greater and greater involvement in medical issues. There had always existed those alarmists who raised disturbing questions about the extent and the intent of medical research in which the government was involved. The movement fueled their concern.

The World War II era brought validation to their concerns. Eugenics, euthanasia, and human experimentation characterized Nazi medical research. Human experimentation and biological warfare research and testing characterized the Japanese effort. The United States engaged in biological warfare research and production and used its own citizens to conduct radiation exposure tests. It also conducted the infamous Tuskegee experiment, in which syphilis infected African Americans were studied and left untreated between 1932 and 1972. Meanwhile, the United Kingdom was also engaged in biological warfare research. Clearly, advances in medical knowledge could have some extremely perverse effects.

As technology increased additional concerns arose over organ transplants and who would get them, how they would be acquired, whether they could be bought or sold, or whether the organs of condemned prisoners could be commandeered. The government and the courts became deeply involved in these issues. Advances in genetic research and the explosive use of DNA has raised considerable concern over the legalities of such information—for employment, for insurance, and for the very fundamental issue of individual privacy.

Medicine, and what medicine has wrought, has become inextricably interwoven into the very fabric of American life and society. And this very fact renders it very difficult to bring about any substantial reform of the system.

That there is a crisis in modern medicine is a massive understatement. A growing number of studies, as reported in the American media, portray a health care system run amuck. Various studies cite the number of deaths attributed to over prescribing of pharmaceuticals, to the misreading of prescriptions, and to the adverse interactions of multiple prescriptions. Studies cite the growing number of "adverse events," that is, medical errors that harm or kill the patient being treated, that are occurring in our hospitals. Prestigious studies cite the prevalence of unnecessary surgery or of misdiagnosis. The figures in these studies vary somewhat, but they are consistently alarming.

Enter Iatrogenic Medicine

Articles in *The Journal of the American Medical Association* (JAMA), and *The New England Journal of Medicine,* both highly respected peer reviewed professional journals, as reported by such well received organizations such as the Institute of Medicine, a unit of the National Academy of Science, have joined in on the chorus of concern. Data has been released that attributes up to 100,000 deaths each year to hospital error, a like amount for various miscues associated with the use of pharmaceuticals, and most recently (July, 2000, an article in JAMA that suggests that 250,000 deaths each year are caused by the medical system. This number of deaths from any other cause would be deemed an epidemic.

Such deaths are referred to as "iatrogenic," meaning that they are the direct result of a medical treatment or intervention. Untreated, it is quite possible that that patient would have eventually died from the condition being treated, but it was the treatment, and not the disease, that brought about the immediate fatal circumstances.

As shocking as these figures are, they are far from being totally accurate. They are based on reported incidents, usually occurring in an institutional setting. Most reporting mechanisms are voluntary. Individuals and institutions do not voluntarily report information that might make them subject to a lawsuit. Further, the data does not reflect causes of death that could have been attributed to iatrogenic causes because cause of death was either assumed or undetermined.

These figures also do not include information on the number of patients who were not fatally harmed, those who were subjected to increased pain or discomfort, forced to undergo additional medical procedures to correct faulty previous ones, or otherwise temporarily or permanently disaffected by medical treatment. And obviously, not included in the figures are iatrogenically induced conditions that are deliberately kept secret. A serious shortcoming for any organization that upholds self policing to control itself is the inherent tendency to protect one's own, lest confidence in the organization, or profession, or system be undermined. And further, there is a very real practical concern attendant to the issue of liability, particularly in a profession in which lawyers and insurance adjustors are increasingly important players.

Why are there iatrogenically induced incidents, and why do they occur with such frequency? First of all such incidents are not unique to contemporary medicine; they have always existed. Health professionals, in all ages, have functioned within the scope of their beliefs and knowledge, and with occasional devastating results. The longstanding mainstream medical practice of bloodletting was hardly without its iatrogenic consequences. George Washington is alleged to have been bled to death by his doctors. One of the most prominent physicians of the revolutionary era, Dr. Benjamin Rush, was an enthusiastic advocate of bloodletting—the more the better.

Were these bloodletters deliberately attempting to further debilitate or kill their patients? It is most unlikely. They were limited by their own knowledge. Some of the medical practices of the past appear quite barbaric when compared to modern standards. But what will the future have to say concerning our practices. Will future generations look back to the age of intricate surgery, chemotherapy, radiation, and the wide spread use of powerful side effects laced drugs, and judge us as advanced as we think we are? Most probably they will not. Yet every generation is a product of its own time. It would not be fair for the future to judge us by any standards other than our own, just as we must judge the past by its own standards. Some errors are intrinsic to our current level of understanding.

What has made the problem of iatrogenic events so prevalent in the current era is the extensive use of technology. The harm an individual can do, as an individual, is limited. Technology offers a tremendous multiplier effect. One individual can cause tremendous harm with the application of technology, which is equally capable of causing harm in its own right. Technology, by its very nature, moves the simple to the complex.

The more complex a system is, exponentially the greater is the need for control. The contemporary medical establishment is a megalithic combination of medical specialties and attendant referrals, a variety of health care providers, a steady introduction of new drugs, techniques, and equipment faster than the ability to evaluate fully their strengths and weaknesses, governmental regulating agencies, health insurance companies, sophisticated testing centers at one location, laboratory evaluation at other locations, ad infinitum. The possibility for error or miscommunication is monumental.

When physicians made house calls and carried their diagnostic equipment and remedies in their black bags, medicine was simple. Praise or blame, rightly or wrongly, for cure or lack thereof, was easily determined. There was only one medical player with whom to deal. Error certainly occurred; the physician was limited by the knowledge and technology of the day. But the error could not be attributed to the medical system itself

Controlling the Technology

The advent of science, and of the subsequent machine age, brought about a need for progressively more sophisticated control systems. Over time these control systems would increase in complexity, to the point wherein they became an end unto themselves. Machine age, with its need for control, logically leads in to information age.

From the end of the Civil War through the post World War II era, the primary goal of American productivity was the creation of material goods. The rapidity with which these goods were being produced led to increasing problems of coordination, requiring improved control or management systems. This is what brought about the first rudimentary computers. Eventually the controlling mechanisms achieved more importance than the processes they were controlling, and industrial age America was replaced by information age America.

In many respects information age technology is an absolute boon for America. But the complexity or the vulnerability of the processes involved increase the possibility of error somewhere in the process. The telegraph was an amazing invention for its time. All it took was a pair of wire cutters to destroy it. One modern day hacker can create unbelievable havoc. Modern technology also has its vulnerabilities.

The old adage to the effect that "too many cooks spoil the broth," might be well advised. No advancement comes without consequences, and the blessings of modern society might well be the curses of modern society. Yet the types of errors that result from the technical systems themselves are correctible.

Problems created by technology oftentimes can be corrected by technology. Problems caused by strictly human error can be partially mitigated through training, enhanced awareness, positive alteration of work environment, and so forth, but they can also be lessened substantially through the application of something called the "technological fix." A very real positive feature of the technological fix is that it lessens and sometimes actually prevents the consequences of errant human behavior. Examples of technological fixes are seat belts, air bags, and transmission locking devices on automobiles. These devices do not prevent erred judgment or inattention on the part of the driver, but they do lessen or prevent the consequences of the drivers' behavior.

Many problems are correctible. In the recent rash of articles highlighting medical mistakes, an innovation at Brigham and Women's Hospital in Boston has been cited a number of times. The hospital simply computerized its prescription system and patient records. Doctor ordered instructions for patient care must be fed into the system, which then checks for error. In other words quality control is introduced into the system through the medium of technology.

Tragically, the most common form of error in a medical setting is due to handwriting. Most individuals have had the experience of trying to read a prescription they were having filled, and wondered how the pharmacist could possibly decipher it. Scrawled instructions, poor handwriting, and misinterpretation are readily prevented by computer usage. The hospital mentioned above reduced medication errors by 81 percent simply by inputting treatment information into an interactive patient data base.

The process that was implemented at Brigham and Women's Hospital occurred in 1994. Certainly there were monetary costs involved in doing so, but at the same time, medical malpractice suits can be extremely costly. There is considerable data to suggest that, viewed strictly in monetary terms, it is far less expensive to implement adequate control systems than to pay out financial settlements for medical miscues. And this does not even take into account the human factor in the equation. Yet only a few hospitals have implemented this proven procedure in the last half dozen years. Considering the non monetary costs in human suffering, the added discomfort endured as a result of additional corrective procedures, lifelong maiming, and even death, one has to seriously question what is going on in the minds of some hospital administrators.

Acceptable Risk

One of the most astounding mindsets of the modern age is that of the "acceptable risk." In earlier chapters we discussed the growing quantification of medicine as we moved into the scientific era. The tabulation of statistical data has become a major feature of the medical industry, and most definitely, of the FDA approval process. It is most informative to see comparison rankings of health care by nation, such categories as life expectancy, infant mortality, medical cost per capita, and prevalence of certain types of disease. It is useful to know the most common causes of death. This type of information can help guide us in our decision making process.

But quantification has brought about another development: percentages replace people. For example, after publishing its report on medical errors the Institute of Medicine set a five –year goal of reducing medical errors by fifty percent. Various studies over the past several years have all estimated the number of iatrogenically induced deaths to be in the 200,000 plus range each year. Using that figure, then the goal of the Institute is for only 100,000 people to die unnecessarily each year. And this does not constitute the entire story. As we saw above, the number does not include the unreported, undetermined, and suppressed "adverse events" that occur each year. These are human beings, not bushels of corn. If some die from the adverse effects of an FDA approved drug, their deaths constitute an acceptable risk. There is only a problem if large numbers of people die and it becomes public knowledge. This paradigm assumes that there will be winners and losers in the medical care game, and what is at stake are human lives.

When the Institute report was first announced late in 1999, the sitting president, Bill Clinton, publicly called for an end to the veil of secrecy that surrounds medical reporting mechanisms, and asked for the development of better quality control systems for federal medical care contractors. Senator Edward Kennedy, the ranking Democrat on the committee that would deal with such legislation indicated that a fifty percent reduction in iatrogenically induced deaths over a five–year period was optimistic.

Medical mistakes have been estimated to cost the nation $9 billion a year in one report, another $77 billion, and still another $29 billion. The wide variance is in some ways indicative of the problem with medical reporting and with statistical data in general. What is being counted? Some figures include the value of time lost from work, while others limit themselves exclusively to direct costs only. The researchers are free to argue over the efficacy of statistical models. The bottom line is very simple: it is in the billions annually. And even more significant is the cost incurred in human suffering.

Preserving the Status Quo

The medical establishment behaves no differently than any other institution when it occupies a dominant position. It seeks to preserve the status quo, that being the maintenance of its privileged position. It resists change and it is very slow to accept anything new and different, except when the new and different is more than the same, that being more new drugs and more new surgical procedures—new but within the preexisting medical model. The medical establishment touts its scientific basis, yet in some areas it resides in the backwaters of scientific advance.

A medical ethicist at the University of Pennsylvania, Dr. Arthur Caplan, has written to the effect that hospitals have largely avoided the implementation of information age technology. Computerized patient data bases, such as the one at Brigham and Women's Hospital, are practically non existent in the practice of hospital medicine, although they do exist for customer billing. Most medical records and communications in hospitals continue to be handwritten notes and charts. If automobile rental check in can be computerized why cannot hospital instructions? In practically every profession and occupation there has been an integrative adoption of information age technology. Yet as of 2000 one report indicates that only five percent of all hospitals in the United States have implemented a system along the lines of Brigham and Women's Hospital.

It is not an issue of the problem resolving itself; in fact, it is getting worse. Problems associated with drug mix ups are extensive and growing. First of all, the FDA has accelerated its approval process for new drugs. During the year 2000 the FDA received applications for 238 new drugs and approved 98 of them. There were 365 applications for generic equivalents of already approved drugs, resulting in 244 approvals and 61 tentative approvals. This approximates 400 new drug names to add to the list of approved drugs for a single year. This was not an atypical year; while new drugs and generic equivalents are constantly being added, older drugs have a habit of remaining on the list.

The sheer volume of different drugs, the fact that a growing number of drugs with vastly different functions have similar names that might lead to difficulty in identifying them from a handwritten scrawl, and the fact that many individuals take multiple prescriptions, the combination of which might be counter productive and require absolute monitoring, provides a fertile ground for numerous iatrogenic occurrences.

The FDA averages about seventy–five reports a month concerning drug mix ups. The figure means little since reporting of such incidents is strictly voluntary. There are currently at least a thousand drugs on the market that can be confused with vastly different drugs that have similar names. Since very little of this problem is ever reported, the number of individuals harmed by drug mix ups is estimated to range from tens to hundreds of thousands each year. The industry believes that, even though it goes to considerable effort to avoid confusing names, some mix up is inevitable, and the actual percentage of such mix ups is quite small, especially consid-ering the fact that more than 2.5 billion prescription were filled in the United States during the year 2000. The FDA is working on the problem concerning newly introduced drugs, but has indicated that it can do little about the names of older approved drugs.

Many adverse reactions are never reported or even identified. When terminally ill individuals die, the cause of their demise is universally attrib-uted to their illness. No consideration is given to the possibility of another cause, and this is understandable. The complexity of the situation is such that it is practically impossible to even get a handle on the actual numbers involved in adverse events.

As a matter of life and death, literally, patients need to discuss thor-oughly their medications with both physician and pharmacist, what the drug is for, the spelling of its name, its potential side effects, and make cer-tain that appropriate health professionals are aware of all other pharma-ceutical or herbal preparations currently being ingested. On this latter point, although herbal preparations are generally quite safe and devoid of side effects, some herbal preparations react adversely with some pharma-ceuticals. The medical care givers need to know. It would also be wise to have a trusted friend or family member double check the facts. It is not a matter of paranoia; it is an issue of survival.

Who Are the Overseers?

A related issue involves the apparent reluctant, or at least the alleged extremely slow action taken by, the FDA in removing approved drugs from the market when serious problems are unearthed. The issue is buried in economic, political, and professional conflict. A case in point is the extreme reluctance of the FDA to remove the diabetic drug, Rezulin, from the market, in the face of mounting evidence of fatalities due to liver fail-ure. The controversial drug remained on the market for approximately two and a half years. During that time it generated over $2 billion in sales. The FDA later confirmed sixty–three liver failure deaths associated with use of the drug during that period.

It is interesting to note that the FDA employs experts who are on the payroll of the pharmaceutical companies whose drugs are being evaluated by the FDA, to evaluate their own drugs. All that is apparently required to carry out this little charade is for the FDA to grant a conflict of interest waiver.

This practice is probably no worse than medical doctors conducting clinical drug testing trials on their own patients, and being paid by the pharmaceutical companies for their efforts. Is there a conflict of interest issue in this? What is even worse, there have been instances of medical doctors either falsifying the data in order to collect fraudulently from the drug companies, or disregarding the safety or well being of their patients in order to acquire a requisite patient–subject base, or not informing their patients that they are being "volunteered" for a study.

There is nothing inherently wrong with patients participating in clinical trials. Certain rather obvious conditions should be met. One of course is that of informed consent. Another is that the well being of the patient should always remain of paramount concern. And finally the results of the trial should be accurately and objectively reported. It is ethically possible for patients to participate in potentially dangerous studies. When all else has failed, what is there to lose? But again, total informed consent is a sine qua non.

The Office of Human Research Protection, a federal agency which has responsibility for maintaining proper standards in the conduct of clinical trials, has funding for a staff of thirty employees to oversee trials involving over one million human subjects at any given time. Enforcement exists mainly as a potentiality. On a practical level, enforcement generally comes about due to the efforts of "whistle blowers," insiders who cannot tolerate what they see is happening. It appears as if corruption is no stranger to any profession or occupation.

The past editor of *The New England Journal of Medicine.* Dr. Marcia Angell, in commenting on one drug trial scandal that had surfaced, indicated that the behavior of the physician involved, Dr. Robert Fiddes, was unfortunately not an isolated incident. Fiddes was convicted as a result of a whistle blower in his employ. Dr. Angell reported on the television news journal program *Sixty Minutes* that Fiddes was being paid anywhere from $50,000 to $100,000 per study, and the whistle blower indicated that he had conducted 30–40 studies while she was in his employ. As Dr. Angell stated, its is all about money.

Another disturbing story, this one pertaining to the popular impotency drug Viagra, A Maryland ophthalmologist, Dr. Howard Pomeranz, presented a paper in which he pointed to potential serious vision problems, including blindness, that could result from using the drug in certain circumstances. Some individuals already experience constricted blood flow if they are suffering from such maladies as diabetes, and since Viagra acts by constricting arterial blood flow, the combination can so restrict blood flow to the optic nerve that blindness results. The FDA claims it has no information on this issue, and Pfizer Pharmaceuticals has stated that serious vision problems have been extremely rare....meaning what? Whether there is a potentially serious problem here is not definitely known, but there does not to seem to be any great concern to investigate the claim by those charged with maintaining public safety.

Who is protecting the American consumer when it pertains to the controversial issue of genetically engineered foods? As early as 1992 the FDA's stated position was that genetically engineered foods were the same as or substantially the same as naturally grown agricultural products. Thus, there was no need to submit them to any sort of special testing. In other words, the companies producing these foods were not required to prove that they were safe. Suddenly, assumption is allowed to rule the world of science.

Disturbing evidence has been emerging that suggests that genetically engineered food may not be all that safe. A 1998 controlled scientific study in Scotland revealed organ damage and intestinal abnormality in rats that were fed genetically altered potatoes. It seems that the gene added to the potatoes to render then pest resistant, had adverse effects on the rats, whereas regularly grown potatoes had no such effect on a control group. The research results were first denied, then suppressed, but ultimately published in the prestigious British medical journal *Lancet*. Europe is taking the issue very seriously; the American press is unusually silent.

Yet what is interesting is the StarLink Corn issue in the United States during the year 2000. Genetically engineered corn was being fed to livestock, but not approved for humans because it caused allergic reactions. Does this not suggest that there is something in genetically engineered corn that is different from natural corn? Where is scientific objectivity on this issue? The StarLink Corn matter is currently involved in massive litigation. Farmers are increasingly concerned over adulteration due to cross pollination. Elevator operators fear contamination. Food producers and processors fear liability, and Europe bans importation of genetically engineered foods from the United States. Who is looking out for consumer interests?

Government appears to have gone full cycle. Earlier in this chapter we indicated that early in the twentieth century governments were beginning to think of their citizenry as national resources. The motivation may not have been of the highest order (healthy citizen soldiers to fight incessant wars), but at least some rational interest in public health was being advanced. What government agency is wholeheartedly pursuing the interest of the American public today, or, has the citizenry been sacrificed at the altar of commercialism?

Commercialism

The commercializing of American medical care is at the root of many medical problems. For example, an estimated 600,000 incidents of health care workers being accidentally stuck by needles occur each year. Such workers can and sometimes do contract HIV or hepatitis C from contaminated needles. Early in 2001 a television news journal report suggested that hospitals are locked into buying cheaper, but unsafe needles, when higher priced needles with safety features could prevent these incidents. A class action lawsuit, directed against the nation's largest supplier of needles, was initiated early in 2001 by health care workers in eleven states.

We have repeatedly made mention of liability issues and lawsuits in this discussion. It cost money to initiate lawsuits and it cost money to defend against them. Who do you suppose is ultimately footing the bill? Legal expenses are a cost of doing business and are therefore factored into the pricing system. Concerning personal injury lawsuits, those arising out of iatrogenic situations, the legal profession generally receives as fees one–third of the settlement after expenses. It has been reported that the legal costs, from all parties concerned, and this includes court costs, filing fees, and so forth, add as much as thirty percent to the overall annual cost of health care in America. How this percentage was arrived at is a matter of conjecture; it has to be substantial.

It is not only health care that is compromised by the drive for profits. The drive for profits seems to permeate practically every aspect of American life. The added cost for manufacturing a safe product versus an unsafe product, or providing a safe service rather than a risky one, is often quite minimal. Yet it is rejected in the quest to maximize profits. For some period of time house fires in America regularly resulted from faulty kitchen appliances. It seems that such items as coffee makers were manufactured out of flammable plastic rather than inflammable plastic. The production cost savings was three cents per unit. Homes burned to the ground, people died, people were hideously scarred, but in the short term (lawsuits again), three cents of additional profit was achieved per unit.

The American health care system is undeniably the most expensive health care system in the world. It is at least twice as expensive as its nearest rival in the industrialized democratized world. Costs have been justified with claims of high technology costs and the general poor life style choices of many Americans. The data simply does not support this.

Part of the higher cost can be explained by the existence of a two–tiered price–wage system that insulated the American economy during its industrial development. Contrary to notions of laissez faire economics, government has always been up to its ears in shaping the economy, particularly in the enactment of the protective tariff system in 1816. The United States developed in a protected market, enabling corporate America to charge more for their goods, without fear of foreign competition. Some of the surplus wealth filtered to the working class in the form of higher wages. The result was that American prices and American wages were both higher than in any other industrialized nation.

High technology legitimately adds cost to medical care. Yet in a number of high technology diagnostic procedures Japan utilizes them more than the United States. However, the Japanese spend far less on health care, and have a healthier population than the United States. Japan also ranks number one in longevity (when determined by the World Health Organization formula for years of healthy living), and the United States ranks number twenty–four on the same scale.

The argument of unhealthy life style is mixed. Clearly, an overwhelming majority of Americans eat junk food, overeat in general, and lead sedentary lives. These are legitimate issues. But the other side of the coin points to an America with a smokers rate less than half that of Japan. The United States actually ranks well in low consumption of alcohol (number five). And a fair number of people, albeit a minority, are consumed with leading healthy lives. So the rationalizing simply does not hold up to close scrutiny.

An explanation is multi faceted and will be addressed in the final chapter. For the moment, however, one observation can be made. If the United States ranked number one in health and longevity the number one cost would be understandable. But since it does not, critical scrutiny is warranted.

In trauma care, in emergency surgical procedures, and in many of the more invasive medical procedures, the United States is clearly the world leader. In routine medical care there is room for considerable improvement. This is in no way meant to be a personal indictment of health care professionals, the vast majority of whom are dedicated individuals. It is the system of health care that is flawed. It is the incursion of commercial and special interest decision making in the realm that should be the domain of the health professional that is flawed. It is the mindset of treating disease rather than maintaining health that needs to be reprioritized. These, and a number of other issues will be discussed in the final chapter.

Chapter Summary

- Modern medicine has achieved numerous successes, but they have not come without a price.
- There is a significant credibility issue with the American medico-industrial complex and its government partner.
- The modern nation-state moved into health care issues to legitimatize itself, establish a medical monopoly, and curtail freedom of choice.
- Medicine has become intertwined with government and commerce, raising questions of conflict of interest.
- National concern with health issues was partly due to high rejection rates of draftees for health reasons.
- European nations "socialized" their health care systems. Socialism was equated with communism in the United States and was rejected. American health care remains market driven.
- Private health insurance plans constitute the preferred mode of payment for health care in America.

- There is considerable evidence to the effect that many governments have engaged in medical research for the most perverse reasons.
- The term "iatrogenic" refers to harm or death resulting from medical treatment or intervention.
- As long as there has been medical treatment there has been iatrogenic events. George Washington was bled to death by his physicians.
- The number of iatrogenic events, as reported by prestigious sources, has reached epidemic proportions.
- The practice of medicine at any period of time is limited by its current knowledge base and prevailing paradigm.
- Complexity of the delivery system, extensive use of technology, and chemical medicine greatly increase of the chance for an iatrogenic event.
- Many problems associated with high technology can be lessened with a "technological fix." Many "fixes" are quite simple. Why are they not being widely implemented?
- The concept of "acceptable risk" is both impersonal and dehumanizing.
- The economic cost of medical mistakes is staggering—far more than the cost of implementing quality control systems.
- Information age technology is used less in the medical industry than most other industries.
- Due to the frequency and severity of pharmaceutical mix-ups, the health care consumer must be well informed concerning their prescriptions. It literally is a matter of life and death.
- The FDA has approved a number of drugs that had disastrous effects. It appears to some that the FDA is very slow in recalling dangerous drugs from the market.

- There is considerable evidence that commercialism dominates the medical industry.
- At issue is who is championing the cause of the consumer concerning genetically engineered foods?
- Legal expenses account for a growing percentage of the health care dollar.
- The American health care system is the most expensive in the world, at least twice that of any other nation.
- The United States ranks low compared to other industrialized democracies in most health care categories.
- In trauma care the United States is clearly number one.
- Commercialism and dogmatism dominate American health care.
- It is the health care delivery system that is mostly to blame for America's medical fiasco.

Chapter Nine

A New Medical Paradigm

In the preceding chapter the crisis in modern medicine was discussed. Since the crisis status of modern medicine was being discussed, emphasis was on what was wrong with modern medicine. However, not everything is wrong with medicine. There have been many positive achievements, and these achievements provide a solid foundation for the medicine of the future.

Let us begin this chapter by discussing those aspects of existing medical practice that should be maintained and enhanced. Next we will discuss those practices or systems that should be discarded. Finally, we will speculate on the "new medicine" of the future.

This material is subjective. As has been emphasized throughout this work there is no "one size fits all" panacea. What might be regarded as a major negative by some health care consumers may work out just fine for other consumers. Specific personal experience may cloud the overall picture. For example, there seems to be widespread criticism of the modern HMO, yet some patients have had very positive experiences with their HMO's. So are HMO's inherently "bad," or is a judgment being made on the basis of a particular incident? Treatment that is viewed as acceptable by some patients may be found intolerable by other patients.

There is a danger associated with proselytizing on what ought to be. The act of advancing a particular approach due to a perceived deficiency may bring about activity that remedies the deficiency, rendering the approach advanced unnecessary. With the passage of time the proselytizers may be perceived as cynical, shallow thinkers, since what they had been complaining about no longer exists.

A problem associated with the study of futurism in general lies in the fact that the very act of identifying a trend or behavior, and then suggesting its ultimate outcome, changes that outcome. We cannot know with certainty and midcourse corrections are a constant necessity. All plans and approaches should be subject to constant reevaluation. Breakthroughs in knowledge occur, public and professional awareness shifts, and definite positive actions might be undertaken. Reality is fluid and thinking must necessarily be flexible.

Goals, on the other hand, are less plastic. The goal of medicine should be, as proposed in this final chapter, humane, personal, affordable, accessible, holistic, and eminently successful health care. How the goal is to be achieved is a highly debatable issue.

Positive Aspects of Contemporary Medicine

Trauma care in the United States is excellent. By its very nature it is quite intrusive, but in trauma cases, intrusive medicine is appropriate. Debating over whether a severely injured accident victim should undergo life saving surgery is not really an issue. Individuals with acute conditions may have placed themselves in the position wherein only powerful pharmaceuticals are an option. Powerful pharmaceuticals do have appropriate uses. Depending on the specific medical situation there might not be any other option.

Diagnostic techniques and procedures continue to improve, with increasingly intrusive and expensive medical testing becoming the norm. Good health is equated with regular testing, and many individuals consider regular testing to constitute preventive medicine. Some tests are harmful and should be considered very judiciously. A number of routine tests can result in accumulated negative effect, such as too frequent x–rays. Common sense should prevail; appropriateness should be considered.

There is the possibility that complacency can come about from reliance on the technological fix. Some individuals believe, that as long as they regularly undergo a battery of medical tests and examinations, with the idea of diagnosing various diseases in their earliest stages, they are pursuing a healthy lifestyle. Dependency on early diagnosis, at the expense of pursuing health, is a dangerous course to follow. It is hoped that Americans are not fooling themselves into believing that they are taking proper responsibility for their health by relying solely on regular tests and examinations, and not doing all the substantive things necessary to promote good health. This is not a condemnation of diagnostic procedures. As has been emphasized throughout this text, treatment modalities should be applied appropriately, and appropriateness is matter for patient and health practitioner mutually to decide

There has been notable improvement in the status of alternative medicine. Some of this may be market driven, but I think there are two basic factors. One, many alternative therapies and approaches are being scientifically validated, and conventional medicine is beginning to blend them into mainstream practice. Two, application of scientific reductionism has led to a considerable expansion of knowledge in the field of natural medicine. Alternative medicine is not reliance solely on ancient traditions; it is alive and vibrant, and is growing as expansively as is conventional medicine.

Another positive development has been the growing recognition of the value of prevention. Conventional medicine is a bit slow in accepting what would be a major shift in thinking, that is, emphasizing health rather than after the fact treatment of disease. The turf battle between germ theory and terrain theory is alive and well. Mainstream medicine reflects positive movement toward prevention as is exemplified by wellness programs, annual "free" physicals, various types of health workshops sponsored by some HMO's, a growing recognition of the value of nutrition, and by the acceptance of some conventionally trained physicians of blended or holistic medicine. Some of the dogmatism is softening.

Preventive medicine, however, continues to reside heavily within alternative medicine. The number of people seeking alternative care each year is growing. Emphasis in natural medicine is on strengthening the terrain: on diet and exercise. Everyone is bombarded with disease carrying microorganisms on a continual basis, yet many people do not contract the diseases with which they come into contact. Even the father of germ theory, Pasteur, eventually admitted to the importance of the body's immune system, but conventional medicine had already embraced germ theory, and scarcely heard what their messiah was saying.

Many Americans are adopting healthier lifestyles. Smoking by adults and hard liquor consumption is significantly decreased. Nutrition and diet programs abound, although some are of dubious quality. Health clubs are found in every shopping center and strip mall, and they are not empty. Despite its poor ranking among the industrialized democracies in national health, the nation does rank quite high in preventive behavior.

What Needs to be Improved

It appears that there are seven basic areas of concern that are in need of significant improvement. The first four to be considered involve global changes needed in the health care arena, while the remaining three areas involve corrections needed within the health care delivery system.

One. By definition a paradigm is a filter or a set of beliefs by which we perceive or interpret reality. The paradigm of modern conventional medicine, by its own admission, is based on an absolute belief in scientific biomedicine. The position is specious at best.

Most definitely, the dogmatism that is so often associated with science (and is actually antithetical to science) must go. Dogmatism is a problem wherever there are "experts" and organizations: in politics, in religion, in academia, etc. Rigid belief is crystallized, encrusted belief. It safeguards the status quo while denying further investigation. Dogmatism is non–science.

The biggest problem associated with the current medical paradigm lies in the fact that it is outmoded. There have been two major stages in scientific development. The first stage made its debut in the mid seventeenth century. It owed its origins to Isaac Newton and his World Machine. During this phase rigid and predictable laws governed the physical world, and the human body was viewed as a machine. Some advancement of knowledge was the result, largely due to the scientific methodology that had been formulated. Conventional medicine adopted the Newtonian model at the opening of the twentieth century. This was when the second stage of scientific development began.

Stage two science is quantum science, the logical progression of the scientific methodology. It looks at a level of reality that is plastic, and one that emphasizes the interrelationship of energy and frequency. In the medical field it is energy medicine (chapter seven). Conventional medicine appears to be, to some extent, locked into stage one science, at a time when the general field of science is becoming solidly moored in quantum science. Modern scientific biomedicine is somewhat out of synch with where science is.

Two. The conventional medical mindset embraces a belief in germ theory, treating symptoms, surgery, chemical medicine, and radiation. It is highly technical, invasive, and monopolistic. There is nothing inherently wrong with much of this mindset—if it is not exclusionary. At issue is how and when to utilize its treatment preferences. It has been repeatedly stated throughout this work that war is not being declared on conventional medicine. Medical care is not being discussed with the context of win–lose or either–or. At issue is what is appropriate, what is truly in the best interest of the patient, and what does the least harm, given the circumstances at hand.

It should be clear by now that some invasive surgery may be the only option for dealing with a patient's condition, and also that some surgery is elective. No issue is being taken with these matters. But when surgery is proposed as the first option, when there are other less invasive options that might work, and when delay for a time will not compromise the patient, then why is not the less invasive approach tried first? For example, the standard medical treatment for benign prostate enlargement is a surgical procedure. Yet there are more than forty published scientific studies in professional journals indicating success in prostate reduction using the herb, saw palmetto. Why the rush to the scalpel when a far less invasive procedure might be very effective? It is the mindset.

It would be silly to argue categorically against the use of pharmaceuticals. Many lives have been saved and many conditions alleviated through their appropriate use. Adverse events, with increasing frequency, accompany their inappropriate use. When pharmaceuticals are clearly indicated, and when there are no viable less invasive options, they should be used. Otherwise, they should not be used. The pharmacy is not a candy store.

Treating symptoms in fine, for part of medical care involves making the patient comfortable, but understand that the treating of symptoms does not treat the underlying causes of the symptoms. Angioplasty and blood thinners are often lifesaving, but they do not deal with what caused the condition. These procedures do not cure anything; they constitute a short–term technological fix. The new medical paradigm must consider the long–term fix.

That there are germs, that germs invade the body, and that germs result in disease in the body, cannot be denied. When the body is suffering from a massive infection, war must be waged against germs, for such is appropriate medical treatment. But equally important is the need to strengthen the immune system so that the need to engage in mortal combat with germ invasions occurs far less frequently.

The modern conventional medical mindset is monopolistic. History is replete with examples of individuals and institutions claiming to be the supreme arbitrator of what is true. Seriously, who dares to claim such arrogance? Unless the government sponsored medical–pharmaceutical combine is ended, no truly substantial progress in health care is possible.

Three. There is a need for official health consumer advocacy channels equal in power to the current monopolistic forces. The stated goal of the American Medical Association is to obtain a monopoly on health care. The Food and Drug Administration has completely endorsed Newtonian based medicine, and uses its power to insure that medicine at the expense of all other treatment modalities. The pharmaceutical industry, for obvious reasons, pursues chemical medicine, and it has powerful friends at court—the AMA, the FDA, and a host of government agencies, panels, and experts, all of which are overwhelmingly within the conventional medical mindset.

The question, then, is who is advocating for the health care consumer? The writings of Thomas Jefferson, and those of the earlier writer who strongly influenced him, John Locke, both emphasize that protection of the inalienable right to life is one of the few legitimate obligations of government. Is right to life being protected by government? Where is the objectivity among the dogmatists who control government policy?

Public funds support the government health care initiative, and public funds support the FDA (as well as funds from the pharmaceutical industry it regulates). Should not equal public funds provide support for a non–biased consumer agency? Currently, all health care information is evaluated within the framework of the Newtonian medical model. The practice is as objective as was that of the medieval church when it passed judgment on Galileo's scientific discoveries according to its prevailing world view. Government funding for research in alternative therapies should be no less forthcoming than it is for conventional medical research.

The number of Americans who have utilized at least one alternative therapy is now seventy percent. This does not seem to represent a massive vote of confidence for the medical establishment.

There should be no doors closed to medical research, especially as applicable to new or promising fields of study such as energy medicine. All approaches and all beliefs should be subjected equally to the standards of truth. The obstruction of the advancement of knowledge, or of alleviation of pain and suffering, simply to protect the entrenched interests of the status quo, cannot be condoned under any circumstances.

Some organizations are fighting the good fight, usually in the courts, defending First Amendment rights affecting the free flow of information. The Life Extension Institute is one such organization. The citizenry is capable of making its own health care decisions without having a government assuming the right to do so in its behalf.

Four. Government has an absolute obligation to its citizens to provide every shred of information it has concerning health care options. Public awareness is an absolute. The boards, panels, and agencies of government are staffed with conventional medicine thinkers, the very benefactors of the outmoded paradigm. Objective presentation of information by government and by media has not been forthcoming.

Tax dollars support the government's medical information sites. Yet an article in *The Journal of the American Osteopathic Association*, dealing with just one issue, noted that Medline, the medical database maintained by the National Library of Medicine, carried only one–third of the published scientific studies dealing with a particular natural remedy. As for the other two–thirds, they were available on other databases. It appears as if token recognition is being made of positive non–conventional studies that support the efficacy of non–conventional treatments. In the media this tactic is referred to as selective editing.

The media does employ the tactic of selective editing for most of its news stories. The reporting of the news in America is a for–profit venture. Newspapers, magazines, and television make most of their money by selling advertising. For some time now it appears as if television advertising consists of a steady stream of drug commercials. On the one hand government, with all of its regulation of health care in support of conventional medicine, is assuming that individuals are incapable of making intelligent health care decisions for themselves. But on the other hand, government allows televised drug commercials aimed at convincing the viewer to solicit certain drugs from their physician. When it comes to choices of selecting pharmaceuticals, then they become intelligent health care consumers; for anything else, they are not. There is no consistency here.

Advertising of pharmaceuticals is a major source of revenue for the television industry. Does one bite the hand that feeds it? Are news stories that cast key advertisers in a negative light headlined, or, are they played down or ignored? Is the media part and parcel of the ruling establishment, or is it the non–biased, objective reporting mechanism that it claims to be?

The World Health Organization publishes comparative data on health issues on a nation–by–nation basis. Its data generally does not reflect favorably on the United States, especially since the United States spends more than two times as much per capita on health care than does any other nation in the world. Unfavorable information is rarely reported in the American media. When WHO published a study that ranked Japan first and the United States twenty–fourth in healthy longevity, the study was not reported in the media. Why? If you want to determine how your country compares with other countries on health care issues go to the WHO website. Rarely will you find the information reported by the media.

There are also structural problems associated with the delivery of the news that can result in very negative effects for the American consumer. The media operates within time and space constraints, with television being the most affected, followed by newspapers, and with magazines being the least affected. Televised news items are assembled quickly, abbreviated, sensationalized, and designed to be attention–grabbers. Therefore, they often provide incomplete and misleading information. Take the case of the recent breast cancer drug story.

Evening television commented on a report by the National Cancer Institute to the effect that the drug, tamoxifen, was 45 percent effective in preventing breast cancer in high risk individuals. It was announced as a revolutionary breakthrough (the drug has been around since 1977). No doubt that women of high risk would seek further information, or simply a prescription the following morning. A short newspaper story the day after the television byte, did suggest that there were side effects associated with the drug and that certain precautions should be observed, as there would be with all hormone manipulating drugs. Detailed articles in national news magazines the following week pointed out that one of the side effects of using the drug was an increased incidence of cervical cancer, among other problems. So there seemed to be a trade–off between breast and cervical cancer, with a game of statistical roulette determining the ultimate outcome.

It would seem that before an intelligent choice could be made on whether or not to use the drug all data would have to be available. But those individuals who obtained their information strictly from the television report (the sole source of news for most Americans) were not told the complete story. At issue, then, is whether the story was delivered in a manner that protected a public sense of well being. The information presented was apparently accurate, but did it lead to false conclusions?

In all fairness to the media, however, of all media sources television has the shortest period of time to prepare a story, and the least amount of time to deliver it. Other media sources have more time to develop their stories. The problem lies in the fact that few Americans rely on these other sources. By its very nature television tends to be superficial, and knowing that, perhaps the news editors should take special heed when the story they are delivering can affect the health or even lives of their viewers.

Five. The cost of American health care must be reduced. It is twice that of any other nation, and the explanations given include high technology, extensive use of diagnostics, and the cost associated with research and development. These explanations are flimsy, especially since a number of other nations do the same thing at less than half the cost. Certainly technology, testing, and research are costly, but why are they so much more costly in America?

Fundamental changes in the way health care is organized and delivered have to be made. At the root of most of the cost problem is commercialism. No thinking individual would deny the right of health professionals to compensation befitting their training and skill, or businesses in the medical field making a reasonable profit. These are not the issues. When profits are excessive, when the system allows price gouging, when precious funds are squandered, when cheaper alternatives are ignored, and where inappropriate activities are allowed to continue, these are the issues.

The massive television advertising of drugs is inordinately expensive and is encouraging the nation to become a drugged society. Conventional physicians are trained to prescribe pharmaceuticals; they do not need television advertising to cloud their professional judgment. Advertising is the largest single expense of the pharmaceutical industry. Reducing the advertising reduces the cost and reduces inappropriate use of drugs. Further, the process by which technical minutiae block generics from entering the market at substantially reduced prices, must be changed. Only significant alterations of patented drugs should be allowed to block generic competition, and only for the altered drug.

A number of studies have addressed the issue of unnecessary surgeries, some claiming that as many as 25 percent are unnecessary (this is distinct from elective surgery). If these figures are accurate then the cost of surgeries can be reduced by around 25 percent, and that should lead to a reduction in health insurance premiums and overall lowered cost.

A very subjective issue concerns whether too many diagnostic tests are being ordered. This is almost impossible to evaluate; professional judgment is involved. But it is generally believed that physicians are overly cautious and they may error on the side of conservatism due to liability concerns. If this is true then fundamental changes need to be undertaken on the issue of liability law.

Some studies indicate that as much as one–third of each health care dollar ends up in the legal and judicial systems in the form of fees, costs, judgments, etc. Reasonable limits on liability need to be established, and standardized guidelines and mediation services might help. Juries, too, do not seem to realize that ultimately, it is the consumer who pays for everything.

What is particularly egregious in the legal field is the class action lawsuit, regularly employed against any manner of business or industry. Who has not been contacted and told that he or she is a member of a class action lawsuit, that wrong has been done to them, and that compensation is on the way. Finally, it comes. My wife recently received a check for 62 cents. We celebrated. Last year I received one for a little over a dollar. A few years ago another settlement gave me the opportunity to buy additional life insurance at a reduced rate as my compensation for some alleged wrongdoing of which I remain unaware. Meanwhile, the legal profession is raking in the millions. This needs to be controlled, while fully recognizing the problem of distinguishing between legitimate issues and corporate raiding.

At the other end of the spectrum are the massive sums paid out over health liability issues. Some of this is justified; redress for injury is an American right, and no issue is taken on this point. But what about those gray areas, where scientific proof is lacking or orchestrated fear rules the day? For instance, was the breast implant issue a valid global concern, or did a handful of individuals suffer reactions due to peculiar circumstances, or was panic and fear at the root of most of it? We really do not know, but tremendous sums of money were paid out. And was it not elective surgery, and would not elective surgery be a shared responsibility?

A shift in emphasis to prevention would certainly lower medical costs. Maintaining health as opposed to treating disease after health has already failed, has to be much cheaper. Health professionals need to exercise some "tough love" on their patients. Telling an individual whose life style is leading him to the operating table that he is in good health is not good medicine. He needs to be told that he is killing himself. He needs to know that medicine can only do so much, and that he must assume some responsibility for his own well being. Perhaps health insurance premiums should be calculated like automobile insurance premiums. Then the maintenance of good health would possess an economic incentive.

Using less invasive procedures whenever possible would certainly help to lower cost. The mainstreaming of holistic medicine is an absolute must if health care costs are to diminish. Health insurance companies can help in this regard, and by doing so, they will also be helping themselves. Covering alternative treatments will actually lower costs. This has been the early experience of health insurance companies in California who have piloted the approach.

Since health care is a critical need (Franklin Roosevelt included it in his economic bill of rights), certain of its expenses need to be looked at carefully to determine if they are valid. Many HMO's are currently reporting massive losses, but one need only look at the compensation packages of their chief executives to understand why. The principle of regulation in the public interest has established in America in the 1870's.

We need to instill healthy life style habits in our young people. When did we start selling junk food in the schools? If it was in order for schools to pick up a percentage of the profits at the expense of good eating habits, and ultimately, the ability to learn, then perhaps health conscious individuals had better run for school boards. We need some policy changes

Perhaps the most impossible task of all is for the federal government to get a handle on its own spending. Medicare/Medicaid is a giant sieve. In the absence of competitive bidding these programs pay substantially more to contractors for the same services or supplies that are provided to the Veteran's Hospitals (of course the VA uses competitive bidding). The law was set up to reward the few at the expense of the many.

Six. Inaccessibility to adequate health care is a national embarrassment. In Phoenix last year (2000) a little girl died from appendicitis because her family had no health insurance. Fingers were pointed back and forth, and everyone said it was a shame, but the little girl was still dead. How often does this sort of thing happen somewhere in America every single day? Ironically, the inaccessibility issue is easy to solve. Do all the things suggested under "Costs" above, and health care will be affordable for everyone.

It would be interesting, and shocking as well, if we could determine the true cost of poor health for the nation. Elsewhere we discussed iatrogenic events and their cost to the nation. But what is the cost attributable to poor health resulting from poor nutrition, from lost work, from inability to function effectively, and from various forms of substance abuse? All of these issues affect health care costs, and cost affects accessibility.

A national health insurance system is probably out of the question in the United States. Private health insurance and fee for service characterizes the American health care delivery system. But it can be improved; it can be more humane; it should be accessible to everyone. Somehow, we managed to slip the public education system into America. Accessible to all, with no means test, the free public school constitutes the sole American institution that might be regarded as socialistic. We could move in a similar direction with health care, and we could do so without waging all out war with the god of capitalism.

Seven. Impersonality is the product of the institutionalization of the health care system. A great deal of impersonality is the result of specialization and technology. In the current system the primary care physician refers the patient to the specialist, who in turn refers the patient to various other health care professionals for a variety of tests and procedures. In some instances the primary care physician might be a signature on a referral slip. This is the experience of most people when they enter the health care system, the mechanical model. Take a number and move down the assembly line from station to station.

Broadly trained primary care physicians could alleviate some of the impersonality because their knowledge base would enable them to refer less. Naturopaths, pure osteopaths, eclectic medical doctors, and some chiropractors could all serve as unbiased gatekeepers. Of course, we would have to loosen up on the rigid licensing requirements and end the turf battles. But there are a number of good practitioners, in all categories of health care, who are extremely competent.

A touchy issue concerns the amount of time spent with the attending physician—if there is one (could be an assistant or a registered nurse). Recent studies indicate patients are more interested in talking with their health care provider than what the provider is doing. Most people are stressed when they seek medical care, and five quick minutes in the examining room does not help a great deal. Health practitioners tend to dole out their time very sparingly, proclaiming its value, yet ignore the fact that many of their patients have time that is valuable as well. Health practitioners often forget that they are the employees of their patients, and patients generally confuse the relationship as well.

Perhaps some practices are simply too large. Perhaps some health practitioners need to scale down their patient load. Perhaps a professionally recommended or imposed limit on patient load, one that would allow a certain amount of time sufficient for interaction with the patient would be helpful. Physicians used to interact with their patients. What happened to the "art" of the healer? If the problem is one of shortage of health providers, then open up the closed system and let more in.

There are physicians who do provide personal care, and who do establish personal relationships with their patients. They are health care providers; others are simply in the business. The system itself is not personal, yet it is an established fact that people respond positively to positive stimuli. Is not providing that positive stimuli part of the craft of the healer?

Health Care for the Future

An obvious starting point for an improved health care system is to get the massive bureaucracy out of it. The twentieth century mindset that government and institutions are efficient and effective vehicles for providing service and protection simply is not true. Since they justify themselves by claiming to provide certain benefits (the principle of legitimacy), organizations pretend more than they actually deliver. All government in general is ineffective, yet it remains meddlesome and expensive. Ask yourself how effective is law enforcement, the judicial system, the educational system? Listen to the reasons given by experts for a rising or falling stock market. Really listen. Does anyone really know what he or she is doing? Most decisions of government are based on soft data, on guesstimates, that somehow become hard data when combined and officially announced. Chaos reigns supreme!

It would certainly be a step in the right direction if there was accountability. If all data, with nothing being withheld, were public knowledge, only then could the worthless be identified and discarded, and the valuable be preserved and improved. This may be utopian, for power always seeks to maintain itself and hides that purpose by mouthing altruistic "feel good" generalities. It can be done.

Time and again there are reports on television and newspaper of individuals and groups doing some really positive things in their communities. Then the bureaucrats come with their lists of rules and regulations that destroy what good has been accomplished, and further claim that they are protecting the interests of those whose whom they have just victimized. We really need to get the government out of the most precious and personal and private of arenas, one's right to one's own body.

In the new medical model a thoroughly trained holistic practitioner should be the primary care gatekeeper. The purpose of this individual would be threefold: maintain health, prevent disease, refer when necessary.

The primary care provider should function as a health consultant, sort of a personal health trainer. Personal relationships should be encouraged and appointments should be of sufficient length for in depth interaction. Further, the health provider should function as resource person, recommending behaviors and providing information to his/her patients. Interaction should integrate the body–mind–spirit connection, and whenever appropriate, involve experts in various non–invasive modalities. Patients should be made to understand that, ultimately, they are responsible for their own health.

Emphasis on health and prevention will lessen the need for invasive procedures, and as a result, health care costs will diminish. When the services of the specialist are required, the primary care provider, knowing the patient, and aware of the various options available, will be in a position to make the proper referral. When referrals are made that do result in invasive procedures, the primary care provider should work with the specialist to minimize the side effects of the procedure undergone.

Kicking and screaming the mechanistic medical model will eventually be dragged from center stage. This old model will be replaced by a new model, one that in addition to being holistic, will also be grounded in a new medicine based on energy and frequency. Health care is already in the early stages of this transition. Individuals such as Andrew Weil, M.D., and Richard Gerber, M.D., are breaking out of the conventional mold. Along with others, they are willing to accept the direction in which the new medicine is going. The medicine of the future will be less invasive, because the techniques of the future will be less invasive.

The procedures and treatments of the past will remain in modified form. In the foreseeable future surgery and pharmaceuticals will continue to be mainstream. But long range it will be frequency technologies, and it will be phytonutrients, and phytomedicines that will be mainstream components of the new medicine. It will happen.

Chapter Summary

- Trauma care in the United States is of excellent quality, and is clearly responsible for the saving of many lives.
- Diagnostic procedures are also excellent but there is a danger in relying solely on tests to maintain good health.
- Alternative medicine is gradually being accepted by mainstream medicine, partly because its validity is being proven scientifically.
- There is a growing awareness of the role of prevention; many Americans are becoming more health conscious.
- Dogmatism has no place in the practice of medicine.
- "Scientific biomedicine" is falling behind where science is leading.
- There is a proper place for conventional medicine; there is also a proper place for alternative medicine.
- Conventional medicine must ride itself of its monopolistic goal; other approaches must be objectively considered.
- Government should be totally unbiased in its funding of and its reporting on medical issues. Taxpayers are owed no less.
- Medical costs are excessive and can and must be reduced. Health care should be accessible and affordable to all.
- The impersonality of the modern medical establishment has to be replaced by personal contact with caring professionals.
- Health care must be held accountable. Self policing is often self protecting. Outside monitoring is a must.
- The mechanistic model must shift to a holistic model.
- The medicine of the future will increasingly be energy medicine.
- Much in the practice of medicine is noteworthy; however, there is considerable room for improvement.

BIOGRAPHY

Donald V. Gawronski teaches history, political science, and futurism at the college level and has written three college texts. His interests include a study of change and societal and organizational resistance to change, especially as it affects health care. He resides in Scottsdale, Arizona, where he continues to lecture, consult, and write.

BIBLIOGRAPHICAL ESSAY

The information sources utilized in the writing of this book are many, and in some instances were not chronicled. The intent was never to produce a tome worthy of academia, but rather to provide general information, written on an average level, for the average reader. Footnoting and extensive bibliographical citation were never part of the plan. I drew upon the general knowledge that I had acquired from decades of reading, teaching, and writing, and this accounts for the basic historical theme that is used in a number of the chapters. A number of contemporary scholarly works were consulted; those listed below are representative.

Yet much of the information contained in this book was not to be found in scholarly works, for they have yet to be written. Information came from the websites of a variety of health organizations, both conventional and alternative. The newsletters of many organizations were consulted, but with a definite attempt to maintain balance and to exclude those deemed less reliable. Newspaper articles were frequently used, but only to check back on the original sources from which the articles were derived. Unfortunately, many newspaper articles were not particularly accurate in their interpretation. The same was true for magazine articles but to a much lesser extent. Some sources were openly biased and I portrayed them and the positions they maintained as they presented themselves.

A detailed bibliography of source material is therefore not my intent. For the general history of conventional medicine there are a number of excellent works. I recommend Ray Porter, *The Greatest Benefit to Mankind,*

Norton, 1997. This work is not only an excellent encyclopedic account of the history of medicine, but it also contains an extensive bibliography.

In considering the vast area known as alternative medicine, I used three broad categories of sources. One, I consulted credentialed authors trained in the field of conventional medicine who were also familiar and favorably disposed toward alternative therapies. Two, I consulted credible individuals who had specialized in particular non–conventional fields of medical inquiry. Three, I consulted sources that derived strictly from the alternative medicine movement.

No single work begins to cover the vast and boundless field of alternative medicine, but one comes close. I suggest Richard Gerber, M.D., *Vibrational Medicine for the 21st Century,* Harper–Collins, 2000. Written by a conventionally trained physician, the work emphasizes an open attitude to the myriad of alternative modalities, ancient and modern, contains a bibliography unique to its subject area, and also lists sources of information and organizational contact. Within a similar vein is Larry Dossey, M.D., *Space, Time & Medicine,* Shambala Publications, 1982. This work addresses the impending paradigm shift in medicine, emphasizing "new age," or "alternative" approaches.

Other works in our first category would include Depak Chopra, M.D., *Ageless Body, Timeless Mind: The Quantum Alternative to Growing Old,* Harmony Books, 1993, one of many books written by this popular author. Also consult Terry Friedmann, M.D., *Freedom through Health,* Harvest Publishing, 1998, a holistic approach, and, of course, the two books by Andrew Weil, M.D., *Spontaneous Healing,* and *8 Weeks to Optimum Health.*

In category two, representative of specific areas of health care treatment is Trevor Cook, *Homeopathic Medicine Today,* Keats Publishing, 1989, one of many excellent works on this subject. See also Carolyn Myss, Ph.D., *Why People Don't Heal and How They Can,* Harmony Books, 1997, Robert Tisserand, *The Art of Aromatherapy,* Healing Arts Press, 1977, a classic work, and Daniel Penoel, M.D., and Rose–Marie Penoel, *Home Health*

Care Using Essential Oils, Osmobiose Publishing, 1998. For an herbal approach consult Michael Weiner, Ph.D., and Janet Weiner, *Herbs That Heal,* Quantum Books, 1994. A pioneer classic for its field is Robert Becker, M.D., and Gary Selden, *The Body Electric: Electro–magnetism and the Foundation of Life,* William Morrow, 1985.

For our third category, alternative medicine from its own sources, a good introductory and brief starting point is *Body & Soul 1999 Holistic Health Guide,* pages 90–106, put out by the editors of *New Age* magazine. The article catalogues alphabetically a good number of alternative approaches and briefly describes them. For depth try *Alternative Medicine: The Definitive Guide,* published by Future Medicine Publishers. The group also publishes *Alternative Medicine* magazine. *Disease Prevention and Treatment,* published by the Life Extension Foundation, which also publishes *Life Extension* magazine, is an excellent source, as is *New Choices in Natural Healing,* published by Prevention Magazine Health Books. And finally, *The Alternative Health & Medicine Encyclopedia,* published by the Gale Group, is another excellent source.

Many excellent works by competent authors are now available, and they address practically every field of health care. The reader is cautioned to check sources, and then check them again. Some proponents of particular medical approaches are overly enthusiastic in their claims. This is equally true from both conventional and alternative medicine. Proceed with care, and good health!

0-595-22232-3